The Body You Want

Phil Poole

First published in 2006

Phil Poole has asserted his right under the Copyright, Designs and Patents Act 1988 to be identified as the author of this work.

ISBN 978-0-244-11081-9

This book is sold subject to the condition that it shall not, by way of trade or otherwise, be lent, resold, hired out or otherwise circulated without the publisher's prior consent in any form of binding or cover other than that in which it is published and without similar condition, including this condition, being imposed on the subsequent purchaser.

Contents

Chapter 1	Introduction & Welcome note	p4
Chapter 2	The truth about diets	p8
Chapter 3	The truth about exercise	p14
Chapter 4	The truth about nutrition	p37
Chapter 5	Making the choice	p62
Chapter 6	The food plan	p65
Chapter 7	The exercise plan	p86
Chapter 8	Progress sheets	p114
Chapter 9	Exercise lists & Instruction	p115
Chapter 10	Meal ideas & Portion amounts	p145
Chapter 11	Vitamins & Minerals	p148

Chapter 1

Introduction & Welcome

The fact you have found this book tells me you have been left disappointed and disheartened by all of the diets, quick fix gimmicks and celebrity weight loss DVD's out there, and you're still seeking answers. Well look no further as all of the answers you seek are here within these pages. The truth about everything you need to know in order to take control of your future.

So how are you feeling? Let me guess: you're a little bit nervous and a little bit excited, as this book is the beginning for you. The beginning of your goal, your challenge and maybe even your dream. Your dream of looking great and feeling fantastic. Even if right now you feel like it is just a dream, don't worry you are no longer alone in your quest. I am here to help you with everything you need. I'm going to guide you, educate you and motivate you. My goal has been to devise a way of bringing to everybody what I have done for individuals for years, and that has come in the form of this book. But I know what you are thinking: more diets and extreme workouts.

You couldn't be more wrong! I am here with the simple truth and all of the facts you need to gain control of your lifestyle and ultimately, your body. There is simply no need to diet! My book explains how to do something for the rest of your life and that certainly doesn't include dieting. It is how to lead a healthy lifestyle and how to gain control of your body. It is that simple. Keep reading and everything you need to know, and how to do it, will be presented to you.

Now you may be wondering who I am. So now I will tell you. But I don't want to spend pages and pages talking about myself and trying to impress you, I want to keep it brief so we can get onto the good stuff ok!

My name is Phil Poole, I am an exercise science graduate who spent ten years working as a personal trainer. My mission is to educate everybody about lifestyle and controlling your body. I have heard so many gimmicks and quick fix training techniques and ways to get fast abs and so on for far too long. It has really started to get on my nerves. I know how it feels to struggle to reach your goals. It can be more than dissatisfaction. It can lead to stress and unhappiness and can lead to low self-esteem and confidence. Often people don't understand how unhappy these problems can make you, but I appreciate how it can take over your entire life. But the good thing is I genuinely understand this and feel for everybody out there who feels this way. This is why I have written this book. It is time to put an end to quick fixes and money making gimmicks and together we will achieve *'the body you want'*.

I have spent what feels like a lifetime researching and teaching nutrition and training techniques, and I have tried all of the ideas out there. This book is the conclusion that I have come to. This is the truth about all aspects of exercise and nutrition that you will need to know, and it is also easily sustainable. If this book enabled you to achieve results but was not sustainable it would still sell for sure. But that is not good enough for me, and it should not be good enough for you either. I want it to be achievable and sustainable for everybody and not just for a few weeks or months but for the rest of your lives. I don't want to make a fast quid, I want to educate the nation and build a healthier population, and to help all of you who suffer with a lack of confidence and self-esteem because of your body, because we can change it. Everybody can improve on what they have right now; we can always make progress and reach potential. Together we can change your lives. And there is no better time to start than right now, so without any further ado let's get right to the facts and begin with the truth about diets.

Chapter 2

The truth about diets

Now this is the part of my book which many of you may turn to first expecting to find that secret hidden formula for dieting. Well I am sorry to disappoint you but this is just some plain old diet truth. You may be thinking im not interested in fancy scientific explanations I just want the simple answer, well that's exactly what I am going to do, give you the simple answer.

Many of you may have tried the odd diet in the past, some of you may be thinking of trying one, and others may have tried every diet there is to try. Now for those of you who have tried diets, you may not like this next part. Even if you managed to lose weight on your diet it still hasn't worked. Now let me explain this before you get upset with me. There are two problems with diets. Firstly, and the smaller of the two problems, is that you can lose weight but relatively little fat. You may be asking how? I will come to that explanation in just a minute. The second problem is the larger problem, and im going to explain this problem first.

The problem with a diet is that very often you do not eat enough calories, hence the reason for the weight loss. I hear some of you say how is that a problem? Well this causes two further problems. Firstly this is unsustainable, so therefore it can only be a short term goal. So where do you go from here? Do you give up or start a new diet? The second problem is that by lowering your calorie intake by extreme amounts, very often your body will not have enough calories to carry out basic functions and for energy. The result of this is a process called glyconeogenesis... I know I said I would keep this simple! This basically means that when your body runs out of energy (carbohydrate) it uses muscle (protein) and turns it into energy or carbohydrate. Now by using this muscle you will see a rapid drop in weight, usually seen at the start of the diet. This is because muscle is dense and weighs a lot, and also contains water, so there is further weight loss in the form of the stored water. Now on the scales this looks very pleasing and makes you happy... briefly! But I want more than that. I want you to be happy period. Now back to my explanation. The problem with losing muscle (or using it for energy) is the slowing down of the metabolic rate. This simply means that your body needs less calories than it did before to sustain itself. The amount of muscle (active tissue) that you have affects how many calories your body needs. Therefore, the less muscle you have; the fewer calories your body will need. The good news is that if you have dieted, even extremely, this effect is reversible. It may just take a short while longer to get the results you want, but the answers you need are all coming up in the next few chapters so you don't need to worry.

Now this drop in muscle, and therefore metabolic rate (how many calories the body needs), explains why normally, after a couple of weeks, the diet has stopped working so well or has stopped working at all. You hit the wall so to speak. You have lowered the calorie needs of the body, by using the muscle as energy, until it can now sustain itself on the amount of calories that you are eating on your diet. Now this may seem a little unfair: all that hard work and calorie counting and ultimately it has put you back a few weeks on your target. But don't give up! I am with you on this, and all the help to put things right is here. You may well be feeling a little bit like, *yes that did happen to me*, and also a little bit angry that the diets don't explain this. People normally feel like the penny has just dropped and that now it all seems to make sense. But that is now all in the past; the only thing you can do is to take the positive from your experience. At least now you know you have what it takes to follow a plan, reach goals and succeed. That is the hardest part, now you have already begun on your road to success. You should give yourself a pat on the back for that. Now that you have the correct information imagine what you can achieve.

Commonly, the next stage on the diet would be to give in, it's stopped working, your hungry, frustrated and low on energy. Somebody next to you is looking great and eating a chocolate muffin and drinking cappuccino, it's not fair! Well you're right, genetics can play a big role, but when you learn all the facts, you can achieve all that you want as well.

So you give up the diet and start to eat normally again, losing those hunger pains feels good. But now what happens? You actually gain more weight. How is this possible? You knew you would lose no more weight but you shouldn't gain weight, surely your not eating too much. Well, remember that by losing weight on your diet you have actually lost a lot of the active tissue (muscle), so your body now needs less calories than before which means, yes that's right, your body now gains weight easier than before. I've heard many of you say, I only have to look at that piece of cake and it goes straight to my thighs. Well things aren't quite that bad but I know how you feel. I've always had a love for pizza, especially cold from the fridge, and you know what, I still eat it. You can eat all the foods that you love too when you have read my food plan and when you know the right times to eat certain foods and what quantities are good for us. All you have to do is keep reading.

OK, so your diet has stopped working, you have a decision to make. You are gaining weight, what do you do now? Often what happens is that people try the next diet, or the same diet more intensely, but the same scenario repeats itself. Now eventually this can lead to problems with losing too much body weight such as those seen with eating disorders, but for most people the hunger pains become too much. This is where the term yo-yo dieting comes from, gaining and losing weight in this manner.

So here is the trick, that secret bit of information that you have been searching for. Stop dieting! You can eat more food than you think, just the right food. Cut out the empty calories (calories with no nutritional value) I will explain this later in the book. You will be amazed at how much you can actually eat and still achieve results: fat loss, toned physique, and on my plan you even get cheat days as well, so you can eat all of your favourite foods. Yes that's right, that's when I eat my pizza. You know what, this means that I don't have to give it up, which means I don't crave it. Sometimes when I have the option to eat it, I don't even need it. In fact, from my experience, this is one of the major benefits from my plan. The people who have tried it aren't being naughty by eating treats so there is no stigma attached to it, if it is not forbidden it's not hard to say no. You have a choice. It becomes hard when the choice is taken away. It is the same with exercise. Somewhere along the way there is a failure point looming if you have no choice. If the program doesn't develop with you and isn't versatile, too many rules increase the likelihood that it will be broken, so we will try to keep them to a minimum ok?

Chapter 3

The truth about exercise

A question that I am commonly asked is what is the best time to exercise? I can give you two answers to this. Firstly, your body will use the same energy to perform a task whatever time you do that task, so physiologically, any time is good to exercise. You will be burning more calories than normal and you will be working various muscles and energy systems. So it is all good. Secondly, the answer that I will give to all of us living busy lifestyles is that the best time to exercise is first thing in the morning, as in my plan. There are so many reasons for this. There are not many people who do not have busy lifestyles: going to work, running a home and having children take up nearly all of our free time. The most common thing to be put to the bottom of the priority list is "me" or you. When do you look after you? Prepare the healthy food, do some exercise, have a hobby. We all punish ourselves like this because everything else seems more important. Now this is normally received with a stunned silence from my clients, because they do not realise that they always put themselves last, and many of you reading this book will be thinking the same thing. It is a simple thing and yet so many of us do it, we don't leave any time for ourselves. Now just because I am pointing this out I don't expect everybody to all of a sudden believe that they deserve more time for themselves, or to look after themselves. So for that reason the best time to exercise on my plan is first thing in the morning. No matter what time your day starts, and im talking to everybody: shift workers, parents getting children ready for school, all of you, you can always get up thirty minutes earlier and go to bed thirty minutes earlier. This is not a two hour workout we are talking about; this is a lifestyle change of thirty minutes per day. If you are sitting reading this thinking well I'm not a morning person, or I have more time in the evening, it doesn't matter. I have been there and tried every scenario, so I empathise with you but things creep in and take priority and you "will do the exercise tomorrow and catch up". No! It doesn't work like that. This is where I have to be tough and ask you to make a commitment to yourself. Get what you deserve: the *'body you want'*. It is your number one priority of the day, of every day, So do it first. Then you can go to work, or get the kids up or even go back to bed and lie in if that was your plan for the day. But I bet you have so much energy and feel so good after those thirty minutes that your jobs for the day will become effortless.

The term fitness can be defined as the ability to cope with the demands of the environment, and that is exactly what you will be able to do, but comfortably. Your day will start with a bang and you will feel great. Now you have to trust me on this, it's been tried and tested, even on me, and it works. Even if the first morning is hard to get out of bed when the alarm sounds, just do it, make yourself. That is the hardest part; it only gets easier after that first day. That is a promise. I even challenge you to prove me right. I want you to succeed. I want you to feel great and it is simple. Forget what you have ever heard or been told, it is all about lifestyle.

Another important reason to do your exercise in the morning has to do with food. If you are eating sensibly, like on my plan, you will have a constant, balanced flow of calories and nutrients entering your body throughout the day. That's right, no more going hungry for hours. If you exercise shortly after eating a lot of energy will come from the food you have eaten instead of your stored energy or 'fat'.

Some will come from fat, but I want you to maximise this with the correct exercise intensity and the correct time of exercising. So exercising in the morning with my exercise plan will maximise this possibility. I will also talk you through what foods to eat and why post exercise and for the rest of the day later in this book

The truth about exercise intensity

A common misconception is that the more exercise you do the better it is for you, and the longer you exercise the better it is for you. So many people constantly watch the clock instead of concentrating on the intensity of the exercise. It would be easy for a lot of people to go to the gym three times per week for one hour, a very popular pattern of exercise. What many don't realise is that just being in the gym doesn't help you to reach your goals. It is what you do when you are in the gym that counts, and if you get that right then you don't have to spend long in the gym at all. Let me give you an example.
Person A enters the gym at 7am before work ready for their morning workout. They spend about ten minutes changing and having a chat with the other early starters. They then enter the gym and spend five

minutes chatting to the instructor and cracking a few gym jokes. Fifteen minutes has passed and they have yet to start to warm up. Next follows a five minute routine of limbering up exercises followed by the start of the main workout: twenty minutes walking on a treadmill at a continuous pace. Person A is managing a full conversation with the person on the next treadmill. Once the treadmill has finished person A goes to the water fountain and has another five minute chat to the instructor. The workout continues in this vein for another twenty minutes before finishing with a ten minute shower having some gym chat whilst getting dressed.

Person B enters the gym at 7am also; already wearing their gym clothes and goes straight into a warm-up of brisk walking on the treadmill. Every two minutes upping the intensity until becoming mildly out of breath and starting to get quite hot. This person then moves immediately onto the resistance machines and does one exercise for every major muscle group in the body. Not lifting anything too heavy but making a real effort on every set. This takes a further fifteen minutes. This person has worked hard but hasn't tried to push themselves dangerously and the workout has taken half the time of person A. Plenty of time for a shower, a bite to eat, and travel to work.

Now can you see the difference here? Person B has done slightly more work than person A but also in half the time, and it is this point that is the important one. It doesn't take hours to overload your body enough for it to start to adapt. This is the key with my plan there is no extra time being spent than what is needed, at the right intensity.

Now I know some of you will be thinking that person B may be fitter, but intensity is the same for everybody. If I ask you to work as hard as you can for one minute, that may be a brisk walk for one person, it may be a jog for another, but you are still working at the same intensity level as each other. On my plan the intensity level will stay the same for all. This is very important because I want you to work to your own level nobody else's. The program will adjust as you do, so if it asks you to work as hard as you can that is always the same, but the fitter you become the faster you will be working. This will seem like the intensity has increased but it is just your body adapting and that is exactly what will happen. The difficulty for you will always feel the same; it will never become too easy or too difficult it will adjust at the same rate you and your body adjust.

The truth about resistance training

Welcome to the resistance training section of my book. That's right, a common fear for people when it comes to exercise. But I promise you it's not so bad, in fact keep reading and like most of my clients this may soon be your favourite part of your workouts. Yes that's right. I am saying resistance training can be fun and the benefits you get from it make it extra special.

Firstly, let me explain to you what resistance training is. It is simply using a resistance to exert pressure on a contracting muscle. This pressure or resistance can come from many sources, weights, dumbbells, barbells, machine weights, body weight or even furniture around the home. Anything else that can add resistance to an exercise can also be used and in any location, for example, water bottles, shopping bags, tins of food etc. So you can see you don't need special equipment to produce a resistance. It actually helps to use a variety of resistances so that the muscles don't get accustomed to one type of resistance. Variety is the key, as with most things, but this is also very important psychologically as well as physiologically. You see if you do the same exercises all the time it can be mundane and you seek variety again to ease the boredom, or commonly you quit your routine. We are going to eradicate this problem with my plan. From now on your routine will be flexible in every way. As long as you work the correct muscle at the correct time, which will be explained in my plan, then it doesn't matter which selection of exercises from my lists that you make.

Speaking to so many people has made me realise how scary resistance training can be. I also know the main reason why it is scary: Bodybuilders. It is true that bodybuilders have very big and defined muscles and that some are very strong. It is also true that bodybuilders use resistance training to make their muscles grow. However, it is not true that if you use weights or any other form of resistance training, you will look like a bodybuilder. If you get the chance to talk to a bodybuilder you should. You will realise that it is very difficult to look like that. 80% of it comes from the food that they eat which is very specific for muscle growth. It would be impossible for you to accidentally look like that from resistance training. The majority of results arise from what you do out of the gym and not in it. It comes down to lifestyle. This is also true for bodybuilders. Yes they use weights, but their diet is very specific and different to that of the rest of us. It is also important the way they use weights i.e. how many sets they do, resting periods, how often they train a muscle group etc. So you can see there are so many variables that can impact results. Now when all these things are changed and the nutrition is different you can expect to see very different results. You can become strong and toned and remain slim and supple. Now remember, this book is all about the truth about exercise and nutrition. The very simple way to test this is to find a bodybuilder, or even somebody that you see who has a body you like, and ask them what they do. If you feel uncomfortable doing that then you can try my plan for four weeks and see the results. I have no reason to mislead you because my aim with this book is to reach as many people as possible with the truth because I am sick of reading fads and money making gimmicks. It is time somebody told everybody the truth and that is my mission.

Now as I've explained already your nutrition is extremely important, as is resistance training. So far we have dispelled any fear about looking like a bodybuilder. Just in case there are any remaining doubts in your mind let me give you a few examples of slim, toned and flexible people that use resistance training: gymnasts, athletes, swimmers, martial artists, and most team sports players such as footballers and hockey players.

Now that I have completely dispelled your fear let me give you a few examples of the benefits of resistance training.

Improved muscle tone

Improved strength

Improved posture

Supports and strengthens joints

Reduces blood pressure

Increases flexibility

Lowers the risk of osteoporosis

Increases metabolism

Now as you can see there are many benefits to name but a few. But before I start to explain these you have to forget whatever you have been told about resistance training in the past because there are more common misconceptions about resistance training. One in particular is that it is boring. The common way it is taught can be boring generally, but remember I am here with all the truths. The way to train using resistance on my plan is very exciting and fun. So erase from your mind what you have been told in the past and continue reading with anticipation for the way I am going to teach it to you. You will be surprised and you may even have more fun than you expected with my workouts. In fact there will be no time to get bored.

I'm now going to explain some of those benefits to you, some of the ones you may not understand or possibly not even heard of. I normally ask my clients what they know about something we do, and the usual response given to resistance training is that it makes the muscles bigger and stronger. Muscle tone is also a common response. But what about the others? There are six more on the list, important benefits that I will now explain:

(a) Improved posture- Now this is closely connected to strength of joints. When all parts of the body are worked equally, like in my plan, all of the joints are also strengthened which gives support throughout the body. This means that all of the joints are working through their correct planes of movement and are not unstable. You see, each joint has different muscles pulling in different directions. If one of these muscles is far stronger than the others or they are all very week, then the joint easily becomes unstable. Other parts of the body can become problematic through overcompensating for the muscle weakness in the joint. When all the muscles are strengthened, the bones in the joint are held tightly together as they have more support. This also means the spine is strong through the core along with all the other joints. The spine is therefore being helped in line to prevent any abnormal curvature which can be common in weak spines. For example weak back muscles along with strong pectoral muscles can leave the shoulders hunching forward and an abnormal curve in the cervical vertebrae (the bones of the upper spine). So you can see how these two are linked together and the reason why it is important to do some form of strengthening exercise. But also it highlights why you should always exercise all parts of your body to give you balance throughout your body and to prevent a weak point from occurring. My plan ensures that this is one of the main objectives, preventing those niggling aches and pains from becoming more serious problems that can be so common. This is one of the things that a lot of workouts fail to cover. They cover popular goals like 'lose fat' and 'get great abs', but fail to keep your entire body safe and strong like on my plan.

(b) Reduces Blood pressure-Research indicates that regular activity will contribute to the lowering of blood pressure. This is because physical activity helps to maintain the elasticity of the blood vessels. When we exercise, the blood is forced through the vessels more forcefully to supply enough blood to the areas demanding it because, as we know, the blood is carrying the oxygen required. Put simply, the vessels will be mildly stretched during this action and retain more elasticity than in sedentary individuals. If you perform your resistance training in the way described in this book, it will also become a cardio or fitness workout and this will become one of the positive side effects of the program.

(c) Increases Flexibility- Another common misconception is that weight training or resistance training makes you lose flexibility by becoming muscle bound. Now here is the truth. All of your muscles throughout your body work antagonistically, or simply, they work in pairs. Lets look at a joint to explain this (see diagram)

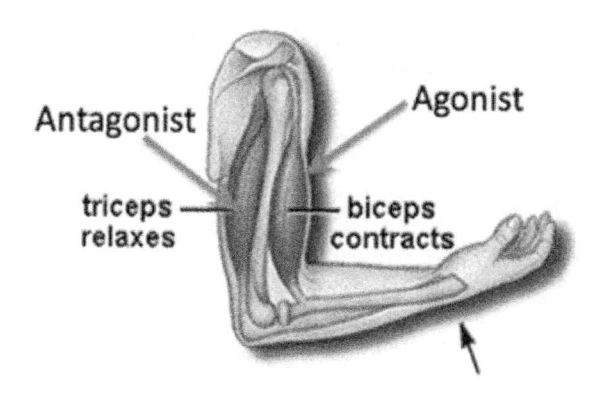

Antagonist   Agonist

triceps   biceps
relaxes   contracts

As you can see the upper arm has a muscle at the front called the bicep and a muscle at the back called the tricep. When the resistance is lifted, the bicep contracts (shortens) and the elbow bends. When this occurs the antagonistic muscle, or the partner (in this case the triceps), extends or lengthens and is therefore mildly stretched. This means that it is constantly being stretched whilst exercising, helping to keep it flexible. Once again, if the whole body is worked evenly then all of the muscles will work in this fashion. Obviously stretching is important and a great way to cool down and relax but resistance training is excellent when used correctly to aid flexibility.

(d) Lowers the risk of osteoporosis- This is achieved through increasing bone density. This is a very complex physiological process, but simply, any impact exercises (exercises that stress the bones), such as resistance training, increases the activity of something known as osteoblasts. These osteoblasts are the building blocks for bone and they are responsible for laying down calcium of which bone is comprised. This activity is reduced in osteoporosis and is especially common in women. So for this reason it is very important to do this type of exercise, and continue a good calcium intake to avoid these problems.

(e) Increased metabolic rate- Just to recap, your metabolic rate simply means the amount of calories that your body needs to sustain itself. Remember when I talked about the truth about diets and I explained that dieting reduces the lean tissue or muscle, therefore lowering the metabolic rate? Well this is the part that does the opposite. You will be improving your lean tissue content by increasing the muscle density through resistance training. This therefore means that your body will use more energy or calories because the lean tissue is active and needs fuel, or in our case food. So the more lean tissue or muscle that we have; the more calories the body needs. There are many other factors that effect metabolic rate such as genetics and age, but lean tissue levels is one of the main factors that we can have an impact on.

So from this you can see that if performed correctly with the correct nutritional advice, resistance training has so many positives and no negatives. As long as you don't decide to push yourself too much too soon, and you warm-up and cool-down correctly as I will explain later in the book, resistance training is perfectly safe and extremely positively effective. The impact will happen automatically and I will take care of the safety part when I give you your guidelines to follow during the workout plan chapter. So now I have dispelled your fears and told you what positives to expect, let's move onto cardiovascular or fitness training.

The truth about cardiovascular exercise

Welcome to the cardiovascular exercise section. Firstly, I want to explain very simply what cardiovascular exercise is. When you hear me talking about cardiovascular exercise in this book, I am referring to your heart and lungs. So anything that gets your heart pumping faster than normal and your breathing rate to increase, we will call cardiovascular exercise or CV. Now you may have heard of CV before. Most gyms use the term CV to describe all of the machines within their facilities that 'get your heart pumping' e.g. treadmill's, rowing machine's, bike's, cross-trainer's etc. Obviously when I am using the term CV or cardiovascular there are many other parts of the body in use and therefore many more benefits. But to prevent this from becoming a complex science lesson, I will be talking about heart and lungs when referring to CV.

Because your heart is a fine-tuned and versatile organ, it has many more capabilities and intensity levels other than work and rest. It can increase from an average of 50-80 beats per minute at rest to anywhere up to 200+ beats per minute during intense work levels. This can be the same in most people. The difference is that when somebody is 'fit' or well trained, it takes a much higher work load for the heart rate to increase. Let me explain this further. The purpose of the heart and lungs is to get oxygen into the body (via the lungs) and pumped (by the heart) to all parts of the body demanding it: muscles and organs. It is carried in the blood and it is used to make the only usable energy source in the body: ATP (adenosine tri-phosphate). If somebody has exercised a lot, their heart will have adapted. For example, it could pump more blood around the body per beat, hence carrying more oxygen per beat. This would therefore mean that it doesn't have to beat as many times to supply the oxygen that is being demanded. This is a very simple process but is greatly affected by the intensity of exercise. Now I have already talked about intensity so let me link the two together. Often when a fitness instructor writes a program for you they will specify a certain heart rate such as 70% of your maximum heart rate. This can be achieved through the use of a heart rate monitor. Now this is all well and good but it starts to get a little complicated and it isn't very user friendly for most gym goers. The reason they will give you a figure like this to work from is for safety and program effectiveness. This is where my plan is different. Through my years of exercising with people I have come to realise when somebody is working hard enough to see adaptation without the use of heart rate monitors. For a lot of people, without guidance, it is very difficult to understand what your heart rate is telling you, so although they are excellent pieces of equipment you will not need one for my plan. You see what I have learned is how best to overload your body. In other words, how best to work hard enough to see an adaptation, without exercising too much or too hard. It is very simple and there are many ways of doing it. Many people I see spend one or two hours on as many days as they can doing endless amounts of CV. The problem is that they never focus on the intensity. If you have been doing CV for a few weeks your body will adapt to that level and then stop adapting. It will just maintain its current state. It needs to do more work than it is used to doing in order to adapt. Now I know that sounds like hard work and normally it would be. But you do not have to do it for a long time. I will give you an example. You can work for one minute above your normal level of exercise and before it becomes too difficult you can drop back to your normal level of work for one minute. By repeating this pattern you will push your body past its normal level and therefore force it to adapt. This is called interval training. There are many ways to do this, which is good because it keeps your exercise varied and interesting. But with my plan I am going to make things even easier than that as you will soon see. I can sense that you are waiting in anticipation! I have a few more things to explain and then we will talk about the plan. The reason I have told you about interval training is to highlight a 'truth' that you do not need hours of CV to lose body-fat, it is simply not true. A saying I always use is that you lose weight out of the gym not in it. The gym, or exercise in general, should be used to transform your body into a fat burning machine. This is what my plan is designed for. It will make your body efficient at burning fat. If you think that you will continue trying to burn your fat in the gym I wish you good luck. Each pound of body-fat contains between 3500-4000 calories (Kcal). You can exercise for an hour and only burn about 600 of those calories. So you can see the battle. You can do the maths, but it equates to a lot of hours spent in the gym to burn relatively little fat. So I am going to make life easy for you. No more one or two hour sessions. Together we are going to transform your body into an efficient fat burner, so that you lose weight out of the gym. After all, that is where you will be spending most of your time!

I feel that I need to highlight another 'truth'. I know that many people will feel that they will have to continue doing their huge cardio workouts in case they lose the progress that they have made. I speak to hundreds of people in your shoes. But I ask you one question: where do you go from here? What happens when you reach your next plateau? Do you add another half an hour to your program that is already two hours long? I don't want to make you feel bad; I want to make your life easy. Imagine having another hour of free time in the day, how nice would that be? To workout for two hours can have a negative effect on somebody attempting to lose body-fat. The chances are you will be eating minimal amounts and working hard in the gym. And I admire your effort and courage, I really do. However, you have been given bad advice, either from an instructor, a friend, or a magazine etc. Remember I explained earlier about diets and I told you about your metabolic rate. That it can be reduced by your muscle level being lowered as it gets used for energy. This can be the same with exercise. If you are working out for two hours and you aren't replacing the energy with food, you will begin to breakdown muscle tissue again to use as energy. The effect of this is to lower your metabolic rate as we talked about. My point with all of this is that the 'truth' is to keep it simple. Follow my plan and see that the only way to lose weight and tone up is to eat sensibly and exercise sensibly. All of the safe and sensible guidelines are here in my book, with a fun and fast workout that will transform your body into an efficient fat burner. I could spend all day or write an entire book about cardiovascular exercise and its effects, but you know what? It is not needed here. I am giving you all that you need to know in order to reach your goals and fulfil your potential. So just like our workouts I am going to keep it short and do exactly what we need to do. So it is time to move on and talk more about nutrition. That's right, food! My favourite part. What's good, what's bad and what we really need.

Chapter 4

The truth about nutrition

Now the purpose of this book is to give you all the tools that you need to achieve all of your goals, by supplying you with all the knowledge you need in exercise and nutrition. There is no point me going into too much scientific depth about the nutrients because you only need to know the basic facts to gain control of your body. Although it is all very interesting, I want this book to explain everything that you need to know in the simplest possible form. The added bonus with this of course is that the book becomes a lot smaller and then you can begin your lifestyle change a lot sooner than if I were to write ten volumes on nutrition.

Many nutrition plans fail because it becomes arduous weighing out food groups and portion sizes and working out your glycemic index and percentages of sugar or fat calories etc. I feel for everybody today attempting to do this because nutrition has been made complicated by the vast array of diets on the market. Although this is all important, it can be made much simpler by following some basic guidelines. So my aim isn't to impress you with yet more science, or with how much knowledge I have, not at all, my aim is to make it clear to you what you need to eat and what to avoid without putting you on a short term diet plan or fast. The idea behind this is that you can eat like this for the rest of your life, so yes, that includes the foods that you love; remember I am a big pizza fan. Once you have learned these principles you can control your body and make the slight adjustments when you need to. You will become to understand what your body needs and when. You will literally become at one with your body. So this isn't a six week diet or a short term goal, this is gaining control over your body and gaining the knowledge you need to know when to eat the foods you love. It's all about balance. I'm sure you've all heard the phrase a 'balanced diet', well that is exactly right. Everything in suitable quantities, and when you know how much you can eat of what foods it is very simple to control. All foods have good and bad points when it comes to taste, nutritional value, and preparation time, and even cost. So there is not one particular food that you should eat every day to control your weight. I get asked this so often, as if there is a mass search for that one key food that makes everything easy. When I know what that key is I can eat it everyday and have control over my body. But it really doesn't work like that, and why should we avoid nice tasting foods at the same time? The missing key is to eat lots of different foods in the correct quantities which I will explain to you in this chapter.

Now the first thing we need to do is simplify the food groups, so that you know what they mean and what foods they include.

Fat

The first group that we are going to look at are fats. Now I can guarantee that at some point all of you have been to the supermarket and looked for the fat free or low fat products. This is ok but it is not the most important thing to look at. You see a low fat product does not guarantee that the food is low in calories. To keep this simple a calorie is a unit of energy the body needs. For example, you may have heard somebody tell you in the past that you need 2000 calories (Kcal) per day. Well this unit of energy is what they were talking about. The food may be fat free but it could still contain lots of calories. For example sugar is a form of carbohydrate and some food may have an abundance of sugar calories but no fat. Therefore you could eat a zero fat diet and still gain fat. Confused? Ok, your body stores calories as fat when it does not need them. Or put another way if you eat more units of energy than your body needs then it stores as fat (stored energy), particularly under the skin as adipose tissue.

Stored energy sounds great doesn't it? But let me tell you that for every one pound of stored body fat there is about 3500-4000Kcals that will need to be used in order to lose that one pound of fat from the body. So when you are in the gym and the machine reads that you have used 100 Kcals you can see how hard it is to reach your target. You could run for an hour and still only burn 600 Kcals. This is very hard for people to hear because it goes against everything you have been told in the past. But let me tell you that you don't have to lose the weight in the gym. The gym is to be used as a tool to transform your body into something that burns fat efficiently. Which means you will be burning more calories throughout the day not just during the time spent exercising. In other words you will increase your metabolic rate, which we will discuss in more detail in the exercise plan later on.

Fats serve three basic functions. 1. They provide the major source of stored energy (body fat); 2. They serve to cushion and protect the organs; and 3. They act as an insulator, preserving the body heat and protecting against excessive cold. So you can see from this that fat is actually quite important. The reason that we need to eat less of it is because every time we eat 1 gram of fat it gives us 9 calories compared to 4 calories when we eat 1 gram of carbohydrate or protein. So because of this, and the lower bodily demand for fat, it is important to limit its intake but not to cut it out completely. It is also important for the immune system, so if you are to cut fat from your diet completely you could become prone to colds and other minor illnesses, unless the rest of your diet contains all of the nutrients necessary, which doesn't often happen. The complicated thing with fat is that there are different types which are generally classed together as fat, and because of that, the more important type of fat is often cut from our diets. I am going to attempt to explain the different types of fat and what they do and what foods they are found in.

The three basic groups of fat are classified as saturated, unsaturated and polyunsaturated. These terms simply refer to the number of hydrogen atoms that attach to the molecule. But like I said I am going to keep this user friendly, so what to remember is this. High fat tends to increase the cholesterol level in the blood, so I recommend that about two thirds of your fat intake comes from polyunsaturated fat. But I will be planning all of this for you later in the food plan chapter.

Saturated fats are found in foods such as:
Beef, Lamb, Pork, Chicken legs & wings, Shellfish, Egg yolks, Cream, Milk, Cheese, Butter, Chocolate, Lard.

Unsaturated fats are found in:
Avocados, Cashews, Olives, Olive oil, Peanuts, Peanut oil, Peanut butter.

Polyunsaturated fats are found in:
Almonds, Cottonseed oil, Margarine (usually), Pecans, Sunflower oil, Corn oil, Fish, Safflower oil, Soybean oil, Walnuts.

Fats are an absolute necessary nutrient in a healthy diet and I will ensure that you get the right portions in your food plan without giving you excess calories that will simply store as body fat. But if you continue to look at your own food labels, the fat contents are generally listed as saturated and unsaturated. So remember, in general, you want two thirds of it to come from unsaturated fat, and if it is listed, in particular polyunsaturated fat.

Water

I think it is obvious to all of us that water is extremely important but it is often overlooked as a vital nutrient. Around 60% of the body is made up from water. It is the transportation system for all of the nutrients and various chemicals, and all of the reactions that take place in the body take place in water. So you can see it is very important. But when it comes to weight-loss water also plays an important role. You see, if you do not drink enough water your body begins to retain water to protect itself. Retained water eventually becomes contaminated because your kidneys can't function properly when you are dehydrated. The liver is then called upon to help process these waste products which then interferes with one of its main functions, breaking down fat. So without sufficient water in the body you can become waterlogged, bloated and obese. This causes problems with sodium. When you are dehydrated sodium can't be adequately flushed from the body, causing further water retention and the whole process is worsened. So you can see how vital water is even for weight loss. It has to be pure water that you consume, not tea or coffee or even juice. Tea and coffee and other drinks contain other substances which can prevent hydration such as caffeine. Caffeine will actually cause dehydration so it is no good to consume water within a caffeine drink such as tea coffee or coke. An easy way to maintain your water levels is to have a large glass every hour of the day. That way it becomes a habit, it is easy to remember 'on the hour' and you don't then need to count the litres through the day. Of course if you are thirsty or are exercising drink more water. If one hour is too long to wait you can have a glass every half an hour.

The next section is protein. But before I get started with protein I just want to check how all of this is being digested (no pun intended)! But is everything making sense? If you have any questions before we go on it may be a good time to read over any parts that you did not quite understand to find the answers you are looking for. When you feel comfortable about all of this information you should continue. Take your time and allow yourself to read parts twice if you need to. Don't put yourself under too much pressure to have a full understanding right away. Remember I am going to be your personal trainer. I will plan all of your workouts and your food plan for you. All of this information is to give you an opportunity to have all the tools necessary to take full control of your body for the rest of your life and to understand why I am telling you to do certain things. It would be easy for me to write a book just telling you what you should eat and how to exercise, but I want you to know all of the facts, all of the truths, so that when you see the next quick fix diet and exercise plan you will have a full understanding of what you are being told and why they will only work in the short term. This way you can understand why it is working, and you will recognise all of the signs along the way and understand the processes that are happening. OK now it is time to continue with the truth about nutrition. We are up to the protein section.

Protein

Protein is used by the body to build, repair and maintain muscle tissue. All of the body's hormones and enzymes are also made from protein. This is very important for you and me and anybody trying to gain control of their body. Do you remember earlier when I told you that you don't lose weight in the gym, but that you will transform your body into something that is efficient at burning fat? Well this is why. You see, the amount of lean body that you have, and by that I mean muscle tissue, dictates how many calories your body needs. So having a good exercise plan also requires good nutrients such as protein to build the fat burning furnace. Without the protein you will not be able to build the lean tissue or the furnace that is going to burn the calories or fat. This also emphasises the need for short workouts. Early in this book I spoke to you about dieting and what happens when you don't eat enough carbohydrate. You will use protein as energy. Which is not good because then it is not available to build or repair the muscle or to sustain muscle. Remember that the less muscle you have the fewer calories your body needs. So this is not advantageous to you at all. The same thing happens if you exercise for too long without replenishing your energy stores. Your body will be depleted of energy and will start to consume the muscle as energy, which as we just spoke about is not a good idea. So the workout needs to be short in duration but at the right intensity, just like the one in my plan. This is another reason why spending hours in the gym is not only too hard to fit into busy lifestyles but is also not an advantage.

Protein is important in regular intervals throughout the day to maintain available levels to build and repair muscle. This does not mean that your muscle will grow like a bodybuilder for example. The size of the muscle is dependant on the amount of calories that you consume, which you also don't have to worry about because I am going to tell you later how many that you need in safe quantities. So there is no need for you to worry about 'bulking up'. You can expect your muscles to tone up and become firm but you would need to dramatically increase your calories to see a dramatic increase in size. I know of course that this is one common fear amongst most people attempting to lose body fat and tone up, because like you, many of my clients have had those fears and along with many people that come into the gym, I believe it is a collective fear which I hope I have helped to dispel here.

I will tell you in the food plan how to monitor your levels of protein. For now all you have to remember are regular intervals throughout the day for your protein intake. You can find protein in several foods listed below:

Eggs, Fish, Meat, Milk, Brown rice, Soy beans, Whole grain wheat, peanuts, White potatoes.

Some of the protein foods are better than others because of the amount of protein in them and the usability of that protein. You may be asking what I mean by usability. Well I will explain that now but don't worry about remembering this because I will ensure in the food plan that all the required levels of each nutrient will be met and you will understand why you need those particular amounts.

Now for the explanation to help you understand:

Usable protein

Protein is made up of amino acids. There are twenty different amino acids that are used to form proteins. Twelve of these the body can produce but the other eight are known as essential amino acids because they have to be consumed in the food we eat. The body can not use the protein without all eight of the essential amino acids present. Foods such as animal products, I.e. meat, contain all eight essential amino acids. Less quality protein such as bread does not contain all of the amino acids. It is possible to add the missing amino acids to this less usable source, in this case bread, by adding another food with the missing amino acids. For example, bread alone has a low percentage of usable protein but paired with cheese it becomes significantly higher. Other good pairings include rice and beans, pasta and cheese, cereal and milk. As I said earlier I will prepare your food lists so that you don't need to remember this because I understand there is lots of information here, but I feel I should include it so that you have all of the facts and truths at your disposal for it if you need them or want to refer to them later.

Carbohydrates

Now for the section I know many of you have been waiting for, carbohydrates. I know that many, if not all, of you will have tried or read about low carb or carb free diets at some point. This is a major selling area in the diets and weight-loss industry, and there have been many published articles about carbohydrates and carb diets, and it has caused quite a stir. I think the best thing to do is to continue in the same vein as the rest of this book and start by telling you all the information that you need to know about carbohydrates without going into unnecessarily hard explanations. This way you will know all of the facts and all of the 'truths' that you need to know, and then you will understand why I am advising you to do what hundreds of people have already done, and that is follow my plan and achieve success. Now throughout this section you will hear many terms which may sound familiar, such as glycaemic index and blood sugar. But like the rest of my book I am only going to explain it in terms that make sense to everybody.

Carbohydrates are the body's primary and readily available source of energy. For the level of knowledge that is important to us carbohydrates can be split into two categories, simple sugars and complex carbohydrates. How quickly carbohydrates are metabolised is measured by something called the glycaemic index. When a carbohydrate metabolises quickly we say that it is very high on the glycaemic index. When a carbohydrate metabolises slowly we say that it is low on the glycaemic index. The speed with which they are metabolised simply means how fast the energy is released. This is why it is always said to avoid sugar. If you eat a lot of sugar you will get lots of energy released very quickly. Now this is fine unless of course you aren't going to use the energy. As we already know any excess energy is always stored as fat. So if you are about to endure some physical activity a small amount of sugar is ok, but if on the other hand you are about to sit at your desk for the next few hours or about to go to bed then it is not advisable to have an intake of sugar. As we have just spoken about it will store as unused energy or body fat. One of the keys to a successful diet is not to cut carbs out but to eat complex carbohydrates in small regular portions, just like protein. The reason for this is because if you eat complex carbohydrate the energy is released slowly and steadily to give you a constant supply of energy without the sudden bursts given to you by sugar. This therefore means that your blood sugar levels remains at a nice constant level.

Now your blood sugar is related to the glycaemic index. The blood is used to transport the nutrients to the areas of the body that are demanding them. For example the muscles when we exercise. If there are too many nutrients they will not get used, and then store as fat. Now when a large increase in blood sugar occurs, like that seen after eating a large meal, insulin is released by the body to lower the blood sugar back to the normal level. What happens then is that the insulin over compensates and lowers the blood sugar too low. This causes you to feel low on energy or lethargic and normally makes you feel hungry again (Red line on graph). With the complex carbohydrates the energy is released slowly meaning that the blood sugar remains constant and never gets the sudden high burst that requires the high insulin release (Green line on graph). If you look below, here is a very basic graph to reflect the blood sugar levels with a complex carbohydrate steady intake (green) and a high blood sugar diet (red).

Blood Sugar Reponse in Healthy Adults

- High GI meal
- Low GI meal

Insulin released (fat stored)

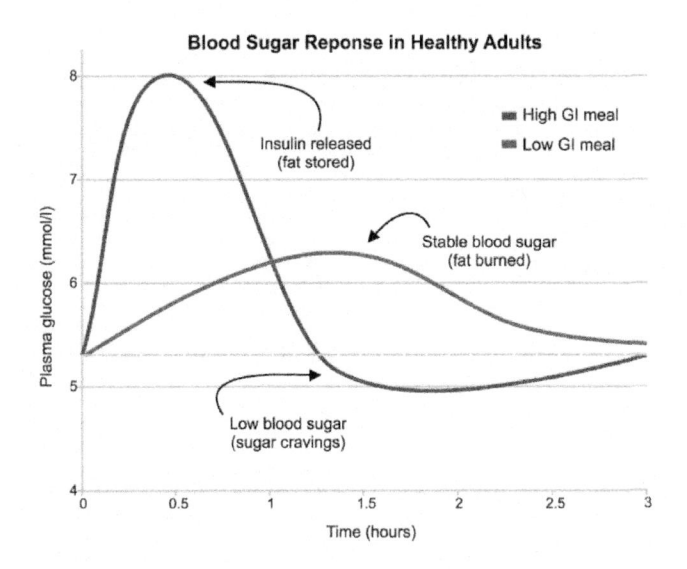

Stable blood sugar (fat burned)

Low blood sugar (sugar cravings)

Plasma glucose (mmol/l) vs Time (hours)

So you can also see by this the reason why it is important to eat small frequent meals to maintain blood sugar level and to prevent vast increase in energy release that when unused stores as fat.

Something else that we have already talked about several times is the importance to have enough carbohydrate available to prevent the body from taking its energy from muscle (protein). If you just eat one or two times per day then there will be times during the day when your body takes its energy from protein because there are no carbohydrates available. This is negative because, as we have spoken about, it lowers your metabolic rate.

Now let's talk about a low carbohydrate or carb free diet using the knowledge that we now have. The first thing that will happen is that the body will demand energy. Like I just explained, if there is no available energy, the body will make its own by using protein to make carbohydrate in a process called glyconeogenesis. By using the muscle you lower the demand for calories within the body because over time, the metabolic rate reduces along with the lean muscle. This is negative because the fewer calories your body needs the less you can eat without gaining weight. However, on the outside this will look like success because when you lose the muscle, or use it as energy, you also lose weight because the muscle weight has gone too along with the water that is stored in it. This process continues until you have lowered your metabolic rate enough to live on the food or calories that you are consuming. After which your weight will remain the same. Whilst all this is happening you haven't lost your body fat, and also you have seen your diet plateau out. So you decide you have done well in losing some weight and begin to eat normally again. But your body no longer needs so many calories because you used your active tissue (muscle) during the diet and lowered the demand for calories. So within days you start to notice that you are gaining weight and become very disillusioned and upset.

Of course all of this is an example, but as a trainer the amount of times I have heard this is beyond recording.

With all this in mind, you can see the importance of carbohydrate within a diet. It is very important not to eat too much of it like all the nutrients but it is equally as important. You may well be sat there thinking well if they are all so important what can I cut out of my diet. This is exactly the point. Nothing! You need to eat some of all the nutrients. This is what is meant by a balanced diet. When you see my food plan you will see that all of the food groups will be represented, no fat free or carb free diets. This is one of the reasons treats like chocolates are kept to a minimum in a healthy diet. Because of the high sugar content, it means that a relatively small amount of food, which often doesn't fill you up, has a high amount of calories. I call these empty calories, calories that have no nutritional value. You would still need to get all of your vitamins and minerals from food in addition to all of the calories in the chocolate. So food high in calories with low nutritional value are best avoided, but as you will soon see you can still eat them at the times suggested in the food plan.

Below are lists of foods that contain carbohydrate:

Potato, Brown rice, wholemeal pasta, Green leafy vegetables, fruits, white rice, Sweet potato, bread, all sugar is carbohydrate.

Some of the foods are higher on the glycaemic index than others but I will give you all of the suggestions in the food plan.

Vitamins & Minerals

Now that we have covered all of the complicated stuff we can talk briefly about vitamins and minerals. I think that it is safe to assume that we all know vitamins and minerals are important to us. The first thing to say about vitamins and minerals is that they are different; they are often confused as each other. Vitamins are organic substances that the body needs and that we ingest in our food. Vitamins do not supply energy they are used to act as a catalyst or a substance that helps to trigger other reactions in the body. Vitamins come in different categories, water soluble and fat soluble. The difference is that water soluble vitamins are not stored in the body so we need to take these on a daily basis. Fat soluble vitamins are stored in the fatty tissues of the body and therefore we do not need to take these as often. Here are two lists for your reference, of water and fat soluble vitamins.

Water soluble

B1 (thiamine), B2 (riboflavin), B3 (niacin, nicotinic acid), B5 (pantothenic acid), B6 (pyridoxine), B12 (cyanocobalamin), Biotin, Folate (folic acid), C (ascorbic acid), A (retinol)

Fat Soluble

Vitamin A, D, E, K

Minerals are organic substances that contain elements the body needs. There are 22 metallic elements in the body which make up about 4% of the total body weight. Minerals are found abundantly in the soil and water of the plants, and are eventually taken into the root systems of plants. We obtain minerals by eating the plants or the animals that eat the plants. If you eat a variety of meat and vegetables you can usually depend on getting sufficient minerals. Minerals play a part in a variety of metabolic processes in the body. You can find a list of vitamin and mineral sources and explanations on what each individual one does within the body at the back of this book. For now though all you need to know is that it is good to eat a balanced diet to get a variety of all the vitamins and minerals. I am going to take care of this for you in the food plan, but I feel that since this book is the truth about everything you need to know I figured I couldn't skip this section, and I know that it is good for you to know why you are doing all of the things that I am telling you to do. When everybody is educated about all of these things and we all understand how and why to do things then gaining and keeping control of your body becomes easy and it can become a very special tool for you.

Now I hear many of you asking what about vitamin supplements? Well the simple answer is that it is ok to use a vitamin supplement as long as you check on the back that it covers all of the vitamins in the correct dosages and if you aren't sure that you are reading it correctly ask one of the shop assistants to help you.

However if you are following my plan you should get a good balance of all of the vitamins and minerals that your body needs.

Alcohol

Most of you may well have a smile on your face now that we have come to the alcohol section of the book. Also many of you may be thinking well I already know that I should cut down or I know all about alcohol. If you are thinking that you are one of those people that should cut down you will be right. The reason I say that is that I am going to advise you not to drink any alcohol during my plan. Many of you may now have a reaction in your head saying 'impossible' I may cut down but I can't quit, I like a drink every now and then. Believe me, I know where you are coming from; it's a scary thought isn't it? A social life based around alcohol is the norm for millions of people; it is part of our culture in the UK. So of course, when I say its time to change something you've known your whole life I understand that reaction. But it is simply a matter of re-educating. Its like this, when you learn to drive it isn't something you question or even think about too much, we drive to work every day, to the shops etc without giving it a second thought. But then one day you go on holiday abroad and hire a car. Suddenly you have to learn to drive on the other side of the car. At first it's a little weird, scary even, but after a few times you realise its not too bad, in fact its exactly the same, it just takes some time to adjust. This is why I am not going to expect you to drop drinking indefinitely. What I will ask of you is for the length of time that you trial my book and plan, also trial not drinking. No pressure. If after four weeks you hate it, you can go back to your normal lifestyle, but I am speaking from personal experience when I say, after the first few weeks of not drinking you will feel great and the awkward feeling when you socialise will be replaced with gosh you look great, maybe I will try what you are doing. Believe me, the amount of people who we perceive to 'love a drink' often tell me I would love to not drink. Well now is your chance to try it. I promise you, you will not be disappointed. You see I have my reasons for asking this of you. Every unit of alcohol adds between 80-120 calories, weather it's a unit of beer or a unit of spirits or wine, the calories amount to the same. There is no nutritional value and all excess calories store as fat. So if you want to trial this book with the continued use of alcohol, it is possible to get results but you greatly reduce the chances of it working and reaching your potential.

I spoke earlier about the effects of the lack of water in the body. Well alcohol will dehydrate the body and have all of those negative effects that dehydration has on the body. Also it places great strain on the liver. Now people talk about wine being good for your heart and/or your brain and all these things. But any positive effect is cancelled by the negative effect on your liver and kidneys so that reason doesn't stand when using my plan.

My exercise plan and eating plan is healthy for your heart not a glass of wine every day. A glass of wine each night will add about 800 calories a week, which many people burn in a week of exercise. So you can see my point. I have to be tough sometimes because this is all of the truths, so I am not going to lie to you all because alcohol is so popular. But as I said before, try it for 4 weeks before making your opinion. There is only one way to fail and that is failure to try.

Chapter 5

Making the choice

Before I move onto the food and exercise plan, this is the part where you get a short break to ask yourself what you want. I have given you lots of information so that you understand exactly what is happening inside your body, and why I tell you to do the things in the plan. If you are very much like me, and memory isn't my strongest asset, then forget about trying to remember everything that I've told you, simply use this as a reference book. You can look back at any section to find the answers to any questions that you have.

But as I said, this is the time to ask what you really want. This is the most important part of this book. Because if you don't want to improve your health and body 100% then this book along with every other plan or diet on the market will not work. You may gain short term success, but if that desire is missing, you will soon fall back into old patterns. So if you are unhappy with your health, level of fitness or body, and on a daily basis you are thinking 'I wish I knew what I had to do to get in shape', then you are ready. If you are thinking that celebrities in magazines look great, I'd like to look like that but I don't like exercise what diet plan can I do, or I'll go walking but I'm not giving up chocolate biscuits or alcohol, then I'm afraid this is not going to work either. I am honest; I am not going to lie to you. If you are not ready to commit to your own life and future then don't waste your money on this book. The truth is this: there are no quick fixes, only healthy lifestyles that provide slow, effective and permanent improvements in health, fitness, fat loss and muscle tone. This book is the lifestyle that is required to feel great and look great. It is easily sustainable. No more quick weight loss followed by immediate weight gain. You will see slow, steady progress if you follow the guidelines and it is simple. After four weeks you will have a full understanding and will not need to continually refer to the book. But all of this will only be possible if you have made the decision. It is no good half heartedly trying parts of the plan, it is all or nothing. Without being fully committed to trying it, all aspects of this plan, you will psychologically not be succeeding. As soon as you have a bad day, without 100% commitment, you will give in and have an excuse. Well let me tell you, my clients give me an excuse, but what they fail to see is they are not cheating me, only themselves. Remember that every time you think 'cheating once will not make any difference, nobody will know!' But you will know. This lowers self-esteem because subconsciously you know you have been weak. It's a slippery slope after that. This is not a food diet; this is easily sustainable, plenty of scope for nice food and treats so no excuse! So what will it be? Have you made the decision; do you really know what you want? If you are unsure about what you want don't waste your money, put the book back on the shelf, because regardless of content if you haven't made your decision 100% then no plan will work for you. That's hard but true. It is time to get committed. If you want to achieve, let's do it! If you are sick and tired of feeling out of breath climbing stairs, Or if you are worn out and depressed from putting so much effort into a diet and you desperately want to improve your body and health then well done, you are ready. Together we will achieve all of your goals, and this is just the beginning, the future is limitless. The only way is up for you, you've made your commitment, now let's begin.

Chapter 6

The food plan

Welcome to the food plan section of my book. I know you have been eagerly awaiting this. My food plan is going to be based around the healthy eating food pyramid. Some of you may be familiar with this but for those of you who aren't, I am going to fully explain the pyramid before I explain my plan and how to use it. I can assure you now it is very simple and easy to use.

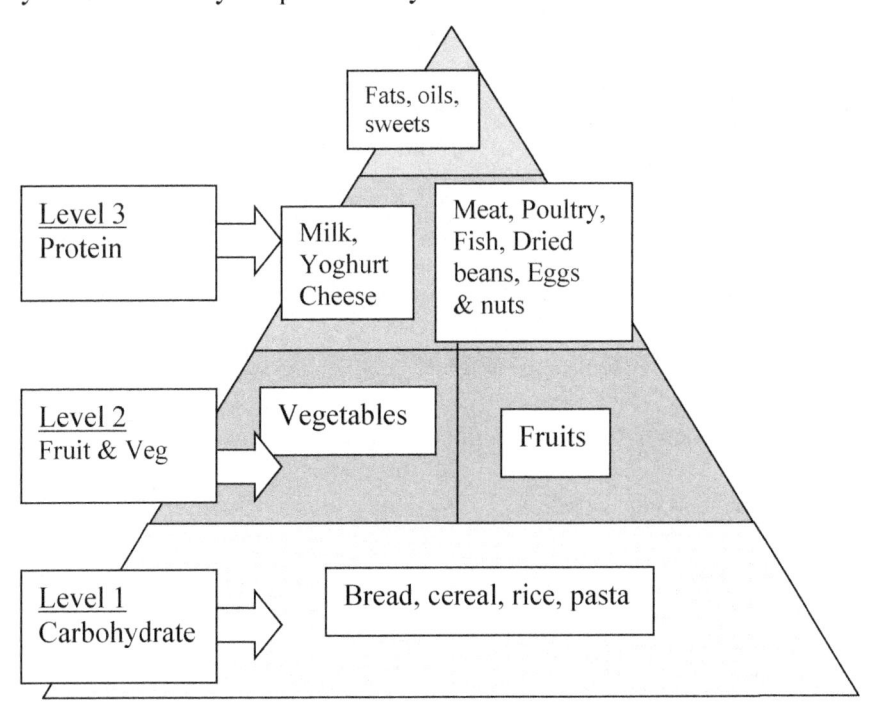

```
                    Fats, oils, sweets

Level 3          Milk,          Meat, Poultry,
Protein   →      Yoghurt        Fish, Dried
                 Cheese         beans, Eggs & nuts

Level 2          Vegetables
Fruit & Veg  →                  Fruits

Level 1      →   Bread, cereal, rice, pasta
Carbohydrate
```

The first thing that you may notice is the serving amounts, and you may well be asking how do I know how big a serving is? That would be an excellent question and here is the answer. These are examples of serving sizes for foods that are used on a regular day to day basis.

Examples of portion sizes (1 portion)

Bread, cereal, potatoes, rice (see pyramid level 1)

1 egg sized potato

1 slice of bread (medium)

1 small pitta or chapatti

1 bagel

3 tbsp breakfast cereal, e.g. bran flakes, wheat flakes

1 whole-wheat cereal biscuit, e.g. wheetabix

2 tbsp plantain green banana, sweet potato, cassava, yam

2tbsp cooked rice, pasta, noodles

2 tbsp uncooked oats or muesli

3 crackers or crisp breads

Fruit and vegetables (see pyramid level 2)

A small bowl of salad (no dressing)

2 tbsp of vegetables

A glass of fruit juice

1 medium piece of fruit i.e. apple, pear, peach etc

1 medium carrot, tomato, etc

6 strawberries

Milk and dairy products (see pyramid level 3)

1/3 pint milk (200ml)

1-2 eggs

Small yoghurt or fromage frais (5oz, 130g)

Matchbox size piece of cheese (hard) 25g

Small pot of cottage cheese or quark

Meat, fish, Alternatives (see pyramid level 3)

50-100g lean meat, fish or oily fish

100-150g white fish

3 tbsp peas, beans, lentils etc

2 tbsp peanut butter or nuts

You can already see that on my plan you don't have to keep on weighing all of your foods or calculating to the exact calorie, the key is to keep it simple. These portion sizes are examples but use this method for all of your foods, remember keep it simple. Using tablespoons to measure food items is very simple.

So now you know how to calculate your serving sizes and you know how many servings per day are recommended it is now important to make this personal for you. All of you individually will have different calorie requirements, different lifestyle activity levels and will all be starting from different body weights. This is the part where you can get involved and decide, using some simple rules, where you start on the plan. Please don't get worried by this; it is very simple, and it is used just to find out how many portions per day you as an individual require. And even if you calculate it slightly wrong it is easy to adjust on a weekly basis without needing to re-calculate. All you need is to know roughly your body weight and also activity level. You can use this simple table to decide activity level.

A: Inactive-   Desk job, Drive to work, Light house work, Make dinner, Walk to the pub.

B: Moderate Activity-   Walk/cycle to work, active job on feet all day, formal exercise in the evening i.e. gym, football, aerobics 3-4 times per week, at weekends cycle or walk.

C: High Activity-   Active job i.e. aerobics instructor, labourer, and workout hard in the gym or sports teams most days.

All you have to do is choose A, B, or C to see which one best suits you and your lifestyle. As I said before if you choose the wrong one it is easily adjustable as we progress.

So now you have chosen your activity level, and you know roughly your body weight, we can easily determine how many servings you require. Remember this is just your starting point so you only have to use this table once, at the beginning of your journey to total body control.

Now lets calculate, using the table below, your serving amounts by choosing your body weight estimate on the left hand column and then move across to A,B, or C which you have chosen as your activity level. This will then allow you to view the servings you require. I have personally calculated all of the calorie requirements for each scenario so that you do not have to worry about calculating it yourselves. You can just see how many servings that you require.

		Activity Level				
Weight		A		B		C	
Stone	KG	Pyramid	servings	Pyramid	Servings	Pyramid	Servings
8	50	1	6	1	6	1	7
		2	5 (3-2)	2	7 (4-3)	2	8 (4-4)
		3	4 (2-2)	3	4 (2-2)	3	5 (2-3)
		Pyramid	servings	Pyramid	Servings	Pyramid	Servings
9	56	1	6	1	7	1	8
		2	7 (4-3)	2	7 (4-3)	2	8 (4-4)
		3	4 (2-2)	3	4 (2-2)	3	5 (2-3)
		Pyramid	servings	Pyramid	Servings	Pyramid	Servings
10	63	1	7	1	8	1	8
		2	7 (4-3)	2	8 (4-4)	2	9 (5-4)
		3	4 (2-2)	3	4 (2-2)	3	6 (3-3)
		Pyramid	servings	Pyramid	Servings	Pyramid	Servings
11	69	1	7	1	8	1	9
		2	8 (4-4)	2	9 (5-4)	2	9 (5-4)
		3	5 (2-3)	3	5 (2-3)	3	7 (3-4)
		Pyramid	servings	Pyramid	Servings	Pyramid	Servings
12	75	1	8	1	9	1	10
		2	8 (4-4)	2	9 (5-4)	2	9 (5-4)
		3	5 (2-3)	3	6 (3-3)	3	7 (3-4)
		Pyramid	servings	Pyramid	Servings	Pyramid	Servings
13	82	1	8	1	10	1	11
		2	9 (5-4)	2	9 (5-4)	2	10 (6-4)
		3	5 (2-3)	3	6 (3-3)	3	8 (4-4)
		Pyramid	servings	Pyramid	Servings	Pyramid	Servings
14+	88+	1	8	1	11	1	12
		2	9 (5-4)	2	9 (5-4)	2	10 (6-4)
		3	6 (3-3)	3	6 (3-3)	3	8 (4-4)

For example, I would choose 12st or 75kg as my estimated body weight. My activity level would be C because I have an active job, and I exercise hard most days. So by looking at the chart I can see that I would require 10 servings on level 1 of the pyramid, 9 servings on level 2, and 7 servings on level 3.

Now if you look at the pyramid you can see that I need to eat 10 servings from bread, cereal, pasta and rice, 9 servings from fruit and veg, and 7 servings from dairy, meat, fish, eggs, poultry, and beans. You can also see that on the chart I have put next to the serving amounts 2 numbers in brackets. They are the 2 sections on that level of the pyramid. For example level 2 has fruit servings and vegetable servings. I need 9 servings on level 2 of the pyramid, and in brackets (5-4) means 5 from vegetables and 4 from fruit.

If any of you are feeling a little lost, don't worry because now I am going to talk you step by step through your own personal requirements. All you need is a pencil and to be able to see the food pyramid and the serving chart on the previous page.

OK, first of all write in here your estimated body weight (e.g. 12 stone). [   ]

Then using the activity level chart select the activity level that best reflects your lifestyle and write it in here (e.g. C) [   ]

You now have the two pieces of information that you require. Using these two pieces of information lets take a look at the overall servings amount chart.

First of all look down the left hand side of the chart to your estimated body weight. Then when you have reached the figure that you have just written down, look across the chart to your chosen activity level column A, B or C shown here by the highlighted section below.

Weight		Activity Level					
		A		**B**		**C**	
Stone	KG	Pyramid	servings	Pyramid	Servings	Pyramid	Servings
8	50	1	6	1	6	1	7
		2	5 (3-2)	2	7 (4-3)	2	8 (4-4)
		3	4 (2-2)	3	4 (2-2)	3	5 (2-3)
9	56	Pyramid	servings	Pyramid	Servings	Pyramid	Servings
		1	6	1	7	1	8
		2	7 (4-3)	2	7 (4-3)	2	8 (4-4)
		3	4 (2-2)	3	4 (2-2)	3	5 (2-3)
10	63	Pyramid	servings	Pyramid	Servings	Pyramid	Servings
		1	7	1	8	1	8
		2	7 (4-3)	2	8 (4-4)	2	9 (5-4)
		3	4 (2-2)	3	4 (2-2)	3	6 (3-3)
11	69	Pyramid	servings	Pyramid	Servings	Pyramid	Servings
		1	7	1	8	1	9
		2	8 (4-4)	2	9 (5-4)	2	9 (5-4)
		3	5 (2-3)	3	5 (2-3)	3	7 (3-4)
12	75	Pyramid	servings	Pyramid	Servings	Pyramid	Servings
		1	8	1	9	1	10
		2	8 (4-4)	2	9 (5-4)	2	9 (5-4)
		3	5 (2-3)	3	6 (3-3)	3	7 (3-4)
13	82	Pyramid	servings	Pyramid	Servings	Pyramid	Servings
		1	8	1	10	1	11
		2	9 (5-4)	2	9 (5-4)	2	10 (6-4)
		3	5 (2-3)	3	6 (3-3)	3	8 (4-4)
14+	88+	Pyramid	servings	Pyramid	Servings	Pyramid	Servings
		1	8	1	11	1	12
		2	9 (5-4)	2	9 (5-4)	2	10 (6-4)
		3	6 (3-3)	3	6 (3-3)	3	8 (4-4)

You should now be able to see the serving suggestions for your own details, so write them in the spaces here:

Pyramid level 1 serving amount required:

[   ]

Pyramid level 2 serving amount required:

[   ]

Pyramid level 3 serving amount required:

[   ]

E.g. my example is as follows:

Level 1 for me was 10 servings

Level 2 for me was 9 servings (5-4)

Level 3 for me was 7 servings (4-3)

Now that you have chosen your serving requirements, you can look back to the healthy eating pyramid and see what you can eat. As I explained in my own example, the numbers in the brackets (4-3) represent the two sections on each level of the pyramid. You can now revert to the serving size suggestions and you will have a very good idea of the size of your portions (see example).

Example of a meal and serving quantities:

> *Ingredients*

1 tomato, ½ green pepper, ½ red onion, selected leaves, 75-100g skinless chicken breast, 4tbsp cooked brown rice, seasoning; paprika, chilli, parsley, pepper.

> *Preparation*

Chop onion, pepper & tomato finely and heat in pan until desired consistency. Season chicken breast and grill until cooked through, boil brown rice.

> *Serving*

Place chicken on top of rice, pour sauce over rice and chicken and garnish with leaves.

> *Daily intake*

2 servings veg, 1 servings protein, 2 servings carbs (see daily requirements).

Now from here it is very easy to gain control of your body and manipulate it as and when you like, following these simple guidelines:

For weight loss:

You are looking to lose about 1 lb of fat a week. If you find that you are losing weight at a speed greater than 1-2 lb per week then it is too fast and we need to adjust the food. For reasons I explained to you at the beginning of the book. It is slow steady sustainable progress that we are aiming for. So the guidelines are as follows.

1. If your weight loss is staying the same after 2 weeks remove 1 daily serving from level 1 of the pyramid.
2. If you lose more than 2 lb per week increase 1 serving on level 1 of the food pyramid.

3. If you lose more than 4 lb per week increase all levels of the pyramid by 1 serving.
4. You can have a level 4 (fats, oils, sweets) 2-3 times per week provided that it does not exceed 200 calories. E.g. 2 digestive biscuits.
5. 1 day per fortnight (2 weeks) you can eat anything you like, provided you have achieved the desired result of 1-2 lb loss per week until you are happy with your body weight.

I say that because it is your happiness with your body that is important. Your health and fitness will be taken care of with the exercise plan so when you reach a desired size, you can maintain your diet using the plan. Simply manipulate it from week to week by making the necessary adjustments that I have just outlined. Remember that muscle weighs a lot more than fat, so don't always be concerned with your weight to the point of being obsessed, it is important to focus on the goals. If you have reduced your size and are happy with your appearance then don't be concerned if the scales tell you another story. This is why it can be useful to measure parts of your body every two weeks or so. This can give you more information to judge the results on and not just what the scales are telling you. Judge it by how you feel, how you look primarily and then how the scales and tape measures read secondly.

The free day that allows you to eat your favourite foods is necessary because as long as you are making progress, this gives you a psychological break and allows you to easily return to the plan. Therefore this becomes permanently sustainable. You will also find that because you are allowed to eat whatever you want, you will not crave it so much because it isn't forbidden at all, and often just a small amount satisfies you. This is when I eat the pizza that I love. But instead of a whole pizza, I find that a slice is enough to satisfy me, and I don't have any of the guilty feelings or feelings of failure that often follow that cause people to quit. I can eat it and succeed, and this is what you will come to realise. It is all about getting that balance.

For weight gain:
1. If you gain 2 lb a month maintain the food plan

2. If you haven't gained anything in 2 weeks, increase level 1 of the pyramid by 2 servings.
3. If you have gained more than 3-4 lbs per month reduce level 1 by 1 serving.
4. If you have lost weight increase all levels by 1 serving each until you slowly start to gain by 1-2 lb per month.

All of the guidelines that I have given you will help you to gain great success in the quest to gain control of your body and get the *'body you want'*. But there are one or two more things that you need to know. The plan wouldn't work if you were to eat all of your servings at one meal in the day. You may well have heard the saying eat little and often. Well that is exactly right. Your body requires energy throughout the day so you need to have regular food intake. Similarly if you were to have too much energy at one time it would store as fat. So the aim is to eat every three hours. This is often a good time to eat fruit portions between meals for example. Therefore on my plan you will be eating 5-6 small meals per day rather than 2-3 big ones. You should never be hungry. This is very important for the plan to work. Too much food at 1 time means fat storage, and not enough for long periods means muscle loss, and as we have already learned muscle loss results in your body needing less calories, therefore less food. So to summarise eat small and often. It's simple!

Another important point to remember is what to do in the morning because this is when you will be doing your exercise. It is important when you wake up to drink a glass of water. The chances are after the period of time spent sleeping without consuming water, it will be in high demand. All of the reactions that take place in the body require water to take place in. So before exercising it is important to hydrate the body. Next, it will be vital to get a small carbohydrate intake to prevent that muscle consumption as it is metabolised as carbohydrate for energy during the workout. This is good in liquid form as it gets into the blood much faster and can be transported to the muscles demanding it. So a sugar drink such as fruit juice or a banana is good.

After your workout is the time to have your first meal of the day. Have your breakfast, and then eat every 3 hours through the day consuming similar serving sizes. Try to ensure that you get plenty of food in during the day, and being careful not to consume them mostly for your evening meal. Like I explained, your body requires energy regularly not all at one time.

Eating out and healthy options.

Eating has always been of the utmost importance for our survival and existence, but at no other time than now has what we eat been so scrutinised. We are placed under enormous pressure by media and celebrity magazines to look in great shape. This takes over the lives of many people affecting even the simple everyday choices such as eating out. This has become a problem because people are following strict regimes and don't want to disrupt that by consuming high calorie take-away or restaurant food. Other people are stuck in that lifestyle, and are trying to make an effort to eat better and to lose a few pounds. I don't want you to give up the nights out with friends and loved ones. And why should you? I have already explained on my plan that you get to eat all of the foods you like on your free days, but here are a few tips to make eating out options lower in calories.

If you choose a fast food option on your free day:

- Choose a burger without mayonnaise or sauces, use ketchup.
- Do not add cheese to salads.
- Try a side salad instead of fries.
- Vegetable thin crust pizza without cheese could be a good option.
- Avoid salad bars, usually loaded with dressings, dips and mayo
- Fish and chips are very high in fat.
- At the Chinese avoid deep fried e.g. spring rolls, fried noodles and rice, crispy meats, sweat and sour, duck and poultry skin is high in fat
- Choose boiled instead of fried rice.
- At the Indian avoid korma and creamy sauces, coconuts, fried or dropped in batter.
- Tikka tandoori, pilau rice and naan are lower fat choices.
- When cooking at home use 1 calorie spray oil instead of bottled oil.
- Steam cook veg, meat, fish
- Use skimmed milk.

- If recipe asks for butter use vegetable margarine.
- Use 2 egg whites to 1 whole egg
- No need to add salt to food
- Use herbs and vegetables for flavours instead of sauces.
- Spend a free day preparing food that can be refrigerated and re-warmed to prevent nit picking at fast junk food.

So you can see from this, the more you think about it; the more aware you become. You will start to come up with your own ideas, but remember these are all just options. There is no pressure with my plan because you know how many servings you are allowed from each level of the pyramid, and how to adjust them as and when you so desire. Remember your next free day is only two weeks away if you can maintain the plan. Have confidence in yourself; I know you can do it. Just stick to the guidelines and you will achieve all that you want. I'm with you on this. And remember, you choose what foods you use as your servings, so you can eat your favourite food everyday provided you don't go over the daily serving amounts and you are eating every three hours. You will find some recipe ideas in the back of the book and with them how many servings they take up. Soon you will be planning your own, and before you know it, you will realise how simple it is to follow just a few guidelines to eating healthy but still enjoying your favourite foods.

Ok, now that you understand the food plan, let's talk about the exercise plan. Remember, eating a balanced diet and exercising equals success. If you do one and not the other, no matter how well one aspect is, you will not achieve your potential. But erase that thought from your mind because I know that deep inside you are a winner, you have got what it takes, you just didn't have all of the facts that you needed to achieve, you simply needed the solutions to the problems. Now that you have that there is no stopping you so let's begin.

Chapter 7

The exercise plan

Through my years as a trainer and during my research into training methods, I have come to realise that all training programs, no matter how precisely they have been put together, at some point become too hard. This is because to increase the workload, as your body adapts, usually means to add more time or more intensity. This is fine but it doesn't allow for any leeway and eventually the program will become too long or too intense. Elite athletes will have trainers with them monitoring every session and realising when a break is needed or what level of intensity to use at particular times. The rest of us neither have the time nor the trainers and scientists to deal with this. Normally when something becomes too hard, something has to give. Either shortcuts are made and the program effectiveness is reduced, or in most cases, the person quits. It is unsustainable. It is unrealistic to achieve and it knocks our confidence; we start to believe that we are wasting our time. It is training for too long without results that can do this. That is until now. What we have been looking for is a plan that is going to achieve results continuously, not just for a few weeks and one which doesn't become too hard to complete or begin to take up too much time. That is why I devised this system of exercise. It is more effective for two fundamental reasons. Firstly, and foremost, its intensity is adaptable. No matter what level of fitness or skill you have and no matter what you feel like on any given day, the program will adapt to you whilst continuing to deliver results. I just mentioned about what you feel like on any given day and that is important. It is another reason why most programs eventually reach a stumbling block. Each day is different and you can't be expected to deliver better performances every single day. Week by week you will improve, but each day is different due to several circumstances such as work, children, sleep, stress etc. So day to day performances will vary but you will still consistently improve weekly.

Secondly, the psychological benefits are immense. Exercise is a state of mind. Often it is the psychological battle that is the hardest; the thought of your workout is often far harder than actually doing it. How many times have you gone home from work and thought, I really don't feel like going back out, I just want a glass of wine and put my feet up. But on the days that you have talked yourself into going to the gym, the exercise part was not so bad after all, in fact you felt good when you finished. It was the psychological battle about actually getting to the gym in the first place that was hard. Well with my plan the psychological battle is always won; you are always achieving. You have a plan to follow but no fail point or minimum requirement so you always win. And being a winner feels great! Imagine doing something where you can't fail. Success is just a matter of time. How motivated does that make you feel? If you were told you could achieve anything you wanted it was just a matter of when, you would probably jump at the chance. Well now is that chance and there is no better time to start. You don't have to wait until Monday… the beginning of the week, your body doesn't know what day it is, and you can start right now. It is simple. Just follow the structured plan coming up and the sky is the limit. In the next few pages you will find all of the exercise information to get the results and *'The body you want'*. At the same time see your physical feeling of energy and wellbeing rocket, and your improved health will be an important and nice side effect to the improvement of all aspects of fitness. You can forget faddy diets and workouts that run you into the ground, and spending two hours in the gym is not necessary. My plan is very simple and it will take 30 minutes a day. You will also get rest days as well. Everybody that has tried this method has achieved a positive result. You will feel better after one week, and by the second and third weeks friends and family will be commenting on how good you look, and after a month there will be no looking back. So the wait is over, let's get to work, you're now ready to begin the program.

The resistance program

Welcome to the first part of the program. In this section we are going to deal with resistance exercise. The first thing that we need to do is to explain what some of the terms I will be using actually mean.

Repetition- A repetition, or rep, is performing a resistance exercise through the lifting and lowering phase one full time.
E.g. a bicep curl from the start position steadily through the lifting phase to the top, and back to the start again by lowering slowly and controlled.

(You can see a full list of instructions for each lift in chapter 9).

Set-	A set is a group of repetitions. For example 15 repetitions = 1 set.

Resistance-	A resistance is anything that can add weight to the exercise to make it harder. For example: weights, the use of gravity, or even items around the home such as tinned food and water bottles.

Failure-	Is when you are performing the exercise slowly and controlled and then your muscles become tired and can no longer perform 1 full repetition.

Cardiovascular- Means any exercise that increases the heart rate sufficiently for a period of time, such as walking, swimming, cycling etc.

Now that I have explained all of the exercise terms I am going to talk you through the structure of the resistance exercise plan, and then to each individual session.

You will be exercising six days per week for 30 minutes. Three days will be resistance exercise, and three days will be cardiovascular. There is an alternative to this plan which involves exercising for 3 days which I will explain in just a moment but preferably this is the format you will follow. So basically every other day you will be doing resistance training. As I said before, your body doesn't know what day it is so you can begin today. You know that every six days of exercise you then get one day of rest. If you stick to the plan, and only if you stick to the plan, you are rewarded with a three day rest every four weeks. Meaning during that week, instead of three resistance days and three cardiovascular days, you will have just two days of each. This gives you time to recuperate mentally and physically. For all the other weeks you will be doing the normal three sessions of cardiovascular and three sessions of resistance. Although this sounds like a lot, the sessions are only very short in duration. If you are finding that you prefer longer workouts but less frequently you can combine a resistance workout with a cardiovascular one. This will mean that you only exercise three times per week but for one hour. If you do choose this option you will spend 30 minutes cardiovascular training and 30 minutes resistance training.

The resistance sessions are structured as follows:
I have split the body into seven major muscle sections. Chest, back, shoulders, front arm, back arm, mid-section and legs.

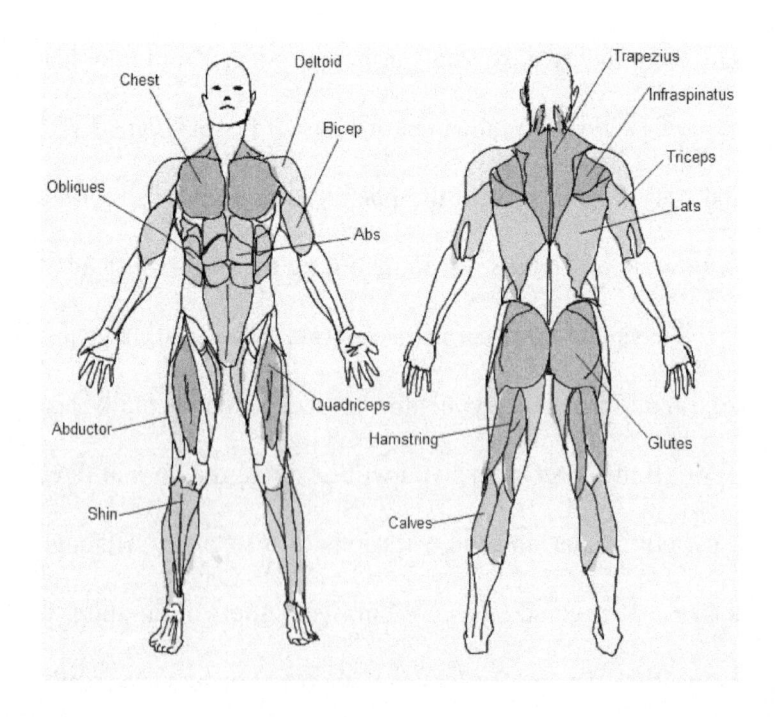

Each of these groups will be worked during each resistance session, and they will all be worked by choosing one exercise from the exercise lists (see chapter 9) for each group. This gives you a total of seven exercises per session. This means that each session will give you an opportunity to try new exercises, and also to prevent your body from adapting to what you are doing. So for example, I am going to choose one exercise from the list for each muscle area of the body that I have just explained to you, and they are listed below to give you an example of one possible routine for your resistance day.

Chest- Dumbbell press

Back- Barbell row

Shoulders- Lateral raise

Front arm- Bicep curl

Back arm- Dumbbell extension

Legs- Squat

Midsection- Abdominal crunch

I have randomly selected these examples from the lists in chapter 9 just to demonstrate the general layout. You can use this as your first workout or select your own. The key is in the next part. Now your workout should take 30 minutes. If it takes longer, you will be resting too long between exercises or performing the exercises too slowly. But don't worry this will all come together as you practice them. The idea is to do four sets of each exercise before moving onto the next. You will rest between every set but only to get your breath back, no more than 20 seconds. You should be a little breathless throughout but not gasping. You can expect your muscles to get tired so don't worry if the exercises get harder after each set. The plan will therefore look like this when it is written in full (using the exercises in the example above).

Set 1	Dumbbell press	0-20 seconds rest
Set 2	Dumbbell press	0-20 seconds rest
Set 3	Dumbbell press	0-20 seconds rest
Set 4	Dumbbell press	0-20 seconds rest

Set 5	Barbell row	0-20 seconds rest
Set 6	Barbell row	0-20 seconds rest
Set 7	Barbell row	0-20 seconds rest
Set 8	Barbell row	0-20 seconds rest

Set 9	Lateral raises	0-20 seconds rest
Set 10	Lateral raises	0-20 seconds rest
Set 11	Lateral raises	0-20 seconds rest
Set 12	Lateral raises	0-20 seconds rest

Set 13	Bicep curl	0-20 seconds rest
Set 14	Bicep curl	0-20 seconds rest
Set 15	Bicep curl	0-20 seconds rest
Set 16	Bicep curl	0-20 seconds rest

Set 17	Dumbbell extension	0-20 seconds rest
Set 18	Dumbbell extensions	0-20 seconds rest
Set 19	Dumbbell extensions	0-20 seconds rest
Set 20	Dumbbell extensions	0-20 seconds rest

Set 21	Squats	0-20 seconds rest
Set 22	Squats	0-20 seconds rest
Set 23	Squats	0-20 seconds rest
Set 24	Squats	0-20 seconds rest

Set 25	Abdominal crunch	0-20 seconds rest
Set 26	Abdominal crunch	0-20 seconds rest
Set 27	Abdominal crunch	0-20 seconds rest
Set 28	Abdominal crunch	0-20 seconds rest

As you can see there are a total of 28 sets per resistance workout. That means you have about 1 minute to perform each set plus a short rest.

You may well be asking yourself how much weight I should use or how many repetitions should I do in each set. Well this is the key; this is where my program is adaptable and so versatile. There is no specific weight to lift. As I spoke about earlier, due to several factors such as children, work, stress, etc. each day will be different and your body will feel different. But don't worry that is perfectly normal. But this is where the program adapts. You will have no way of knowing how your body will perform on any given day. When you presume it will be tired i.e. if you have had a lack of sleep or lots of stress, you could perform well and vice versa. I have had some of my best workouts ever when least expected. The key comes when you can maximise your workout on good and bad days to reach your potential. To do this you will not mentally choose your level for the day because you could be wrong as I just explained. Your body will choose for you using my method outlined here.

Every single exercise and set that you do, you are aiming to reach between 10-15 repetitions using the correct exercise technique (explained in chapter 9) before your muscles reach that point of failure where they cannot lift anymore. This is very simple. If you reach 10-15 and you can continue then you should continue even if you reach 25 repetitions before you can no longer continue. The aim is to lift as many as you can every time (this is called reaching failure). Which sounds negative but it is actually very positive to reach a failure point; it means that you are doing your maximum effort every time. It is this point that will dictate how much weight or resistance you will use for your next set. Remember aiming for 10-15 repetitions, but you may actually achieve more or less, this is just your signal to change the resistance that you are using. As long as you lift and keep lifting until you can not perform anymore (reaching failure) that will ensure your workout is maximised. So if you do more than 10-15 repetitions you know that you need to add more resistance because it is too light for you. If you can not quite get to 10-15 repetitions you need to take some weight off. Remember that your muscles will be getting tired after each set, so if you do 10-15 one set, don't be surprised if you only manage 8-9 with the same weight the following set. This will be left to your own discretion, the key is to reach failure and as your experience grows you will reach it more and more within the 10-15 repetition range. If you are close i.e. 8-9 or 16-17 then very small adjustments are required but if you manage only 3-4 or more than 18 reps then maybe a bigger adjustment will be required. But this is all part of the fun with your workouts because you will never know how you will perform throughout, other than you know that you will reach a 100% effort each set. It is a good idea to record your workouts so that you can see your improvements, and also if you use some exercises more than others, because if you do, you can then change them to keep your workouts fresh. I have given you a progress sheet in chapter 8 that you can photocopy to use for this and record what you have done. Your rest period after each set can be used for several things. To get your breath back, to drink some water, to change the resistance level, to make a recording. These are all important and you can do any of them or all of them during your rest.

Here is an example of changing resistance levels so you can see clearly what I have been explaining. I am just using the first 2 exercises in the workout as an example; remember we are aiming for 10-15 repetitions when we reach our failure point.

Set	Exercise	Weight	Repetitions	Adjustments
1	Dumbbell press	5kg	22	increase
2	Dumbbell press	10kg	15	
3	Dumbbell press	10kg	11	
4	Dumbbell press	10kg	9	
5	Barbell Row	15kg	12	
6	Barbell Row	15kg	9	decrease
7	Barbell Row	10kg	15	
8	Barbell Row	10kg	12	

From the example you can see that for set one, 22 repetitions were performed. So I increased the resistance slightly. The next three sets I kept the resistance the same because I reached the 10-15 rep range required. You can see that set four was 9 repetitions, but it is the last set of that particular exercise so no more adjustments are necessary. You can see from set six that I had to reduce the resistance because I hadn't quite done enough repetitions.

From this you can see the general format that the plan requires. Give yourself one week as a practice at doing this. Don't put too much pressure on yourself, have some fun, it will become very fluent, just try to smile and allow for more time during this first week. For that practice week you will still be burning up many more calories than at rest, and it is also giving your body a chance to get used to this, so it is still very beneficial for you.

Summary

- Choose 1 exercise for each of the 7 muscle sections of the body (you can use chapter 9 as a reference)
- Perform 4 sets of each exercise

- Rest between sets no more than 20 seconds
- Adjust resistance to reach 10-15 reps per set
- When you begin your workouts, continue to the end without pausing to talk or use the bathroom etc. It's very important to maintain intensity throughout the 30 minutes.
- Record your results

The cardiovascular program

This is the second part of the exercise plan. Before we start on the plan, I want to take a look at a list of activities and their estimated calories burned per hour. This will allow you to see and compare various activities with each other, and maybe see what you have been doing previously.

Activity	**Calories burned per hour (energy expenditure)**
Sleeping	72
Sitting	72-84
Walking (3.4mph)	336-420
Swimming (Leisurely)	360

Cycling (10mph)	360-420
Jogging (5mph)	600
Skiing (moderate to steep)	480-720
Running (7.5mph)	900

The reason I have given you this list is to explain to you that all of these activities will burn calories dependant on the intensity level. For example you will burn approximately 100 kcal for every mile walked, jogged or run. The difference is the time taken to burn them. The key comes when the calories you are burning are coming from fat stores, this is the aim. Remember, there are approximately 3500-4000kcals in 1 lb of body fat. That is a lot of energy that needs to be burned when you compare it to the table for energy expenditure. But it becomes even more difficult if you burn 300 kcals walking, but your heart rate doesn't increase by much. This is due to a very small percentage of the calories burned coming from fat stores. In order to use these fat stores, we need to get your heart rate much higher so that a greater percentage of what you are burning is coming from fat. Now that sounds like hard work doesn't it? Well this is where my plan comes in and it is very simple to use. It is too much to ask for you to raise your heart rate to a high level and keep it there especially if you are a newcomer to exercise. So my plan is designed to be versatile just like the resistance section. It doesn't matter what your starting level of fitness is, you can be a beginner or an advanced trainer, because the program adapts to you. The strategy with this is very simple. I have designed this so that you have three effort levels. The first level is an effort that is just above resting level, for example if you take your normal walking speed and then increase it slightly so that you experience a slight breathing increase and you can feel your heart rate also increase slightly. The second level would be a level that you could only sustain for a few minutes, so your heart beats faster and you become warm and you need to take deep breaths. This would feel like you want to get your breath back and rest momentarily. The final level, level 3, is your all out effort. The hardest you can work, your breathing is fast, you become very hot and possibly sweating. I can hear some of you saying 'that sounds like hell!' Well let me re-assure you, your workout will not be at any of those levels, but a combination of all three. You will never stay at 1 level for a long period until it hurts, that would not be the point. The point is to get your heart rate higher to start to burn a higher percentage of fat stores, but before it becomes too hard you can lower your intensity again. This is designed to get your body into a state called 'overload'. This simply means that you are making your body adapt. Many people will exercise for long periods but never actually get to the level where your body adapts or changes. You can achieve this level in a short space of time. Remember my workouts are only ever 30 minutes long. I have designed it so you will never be feeling as though it is too hard, but you will reach a point where your body will adapt. The great thing is this method can be used with any type of exercise: walking, cycling, swimming, jogging, skiing etc. So you get to choose the activity yourself, you may have a favourite. I am not going to make you do one activity. As long as you use these levels it will work. You can do it outdoors, at home or in the gym. Wherever you like and with whatever activity you like. As long as you structure it like I am about to explain, you will succeed. This is also going to be more beneficial for your fitness because your heart rate will be higher than normal, and it will be forced to work hard and adapt. Working for hours at low intensity doesn't put any pressure on your energy systems or heart and lungs. Therefore, because they can cope, they don't need to adapt or become more efficient. Using my plan will ensure that adaptation occurs. As you adapt, your fitness levels will increase, and your ability to work hard will increase. This will ensure that the program adapts as you do. The structure is as follows:

3minutes at slow pace to begin the warm-up

1 minute at level 1
1 minute at level 2   repeat this cycle 8 times
1 minute at level 3

3 minutes at level 1 to cool down

All that you will need for this is a watch or clock to keep an eye on the time, and then increase your workouts as instructed. The level 3 has to be your all out effort for this to work, but for some of you that may be walking fast and for others it may be a sprint, you decide. But it must be your maximum effort. If you look at the plan that is only a total of 8 minutes hard work and you will be recovering in between during the level 1 periods. If you are a little unsure how to read the structure here it is again in full this time:

Minute	Level
1	Warm-up
2	Warm-up
3	Warm-up
4	1
5	2
6	3 all out effort
7	1
8	2
9	3 all out effort
10	1
11	2
12	3 all out effort
13	1
14	2
15	3 all out effort
16	1
17	2
18	3 all out effort
19	1
20	2
21	3 all out effort
22	1
23	2
24	3 all out effort
25	1
26	2
27	3 all out effort
28	Cool-down
29	Cool-down
30	Cool-down

It will be beneficial for you to change your activities each workout, for example cycle one day, walk the next and maybe try swimming one day. This gives you a chance to use all your muscles in different ways and it will also help to prevent your body from adapting to the program. Remember that your body will adapt to anything that you put it through. So in order to keep improving a change is a good thing. If you only like one activity such as walking, that is ok, you just have to put more emphasis on the program itself. For example, when you are asked to perform at your highest level for 1 minute, you must seek to improve. As you get fitter and your body adapts you will be able to work harder. So your walking speed will increase or you can walk uphill to make it harder. If you can stick to these principles you will get great results. As long as you combine the exercise with the healthy eating plan, you will progress at a perfect rate: slow steady fat loss and improved muscle tone, fitness and well being.

Do you remember before that I told you exercise is massively psychological? It is the same with my plan as with all plans. But there are things that you can do to stay in control psychologically. For example changing the activity from walking to cycling, rowing or skiing keeps your mind fresh. Or if you only like one activity you can do something else to help. You can throw in a changed workout to keep the exercise new and fresh. This helps to keep your mind fresh and it is another way to help prevent your body from adapting to what you are doing. This can be achieved easily and can be done once every two or three weeks. If you feel a little bored or don't change the activity often, you can use a changed workout.

This can be done in many ways but for you, in this situation, you can choose two options. The first one is very simple it is exercising at one continuous level for the same duration as your previous workout, 30 minutes. This does have its down sides because it is hard to stay at a higher heart rate for a long period of time. But a low level workout is ok when being used seldom. It will give you a psychological break and gives your body a chance to rest and recover whilst continuing to burn extra calories. So option one is simply to work for 30 minutes at a level which makes you breathe hard, and try to push yourself as hard as you can.

The second option is to keep the structure the same but to change the time limit of each interval. For example instead of working at 1 minute for each level you can do 2 minutes, 3 minutes or even 4. This gives you longer to recover between intervals but your work intervals are also longer. So this is something you can play around with when you need a psychological break or change. Remember you can do this once every 2 or 3 weeks. If you have been following the plan for a few months and feel ready for a change, then you can do one of the alternatives for a whole week once per month. Remember to continue with your resistance training and eating plan during this period, and always return to the basic exercise plan afterwards. It is also important when changing the routine to maintain a 30 minute workout, no more. It has to fit into your lifestyle as we have spoken about. It is so much more advantageous to work at a higher intensity for 30 minutes and see adaptations occur within your body than to spend two hours at a comfortable level and see no adaptations.

Now you may have noticed that in this section I have not talked about warming up, stretching or cooling down. I am now going to explain this and my reasons for not including it so far.

For those of you who have been to a gym before, you may well have been given a series of stretches to do as part of a warm-up. In my plan you will not do that. The reason for this is because your muscles especially at the core are not warm enough to be stretched before a workout and the resulting effect will be small tears to the muscle fibres. It is very important to stretch and remain flexible, but this should be done at the end of your workout as part of your cool down. Now you will find a list of stretches with diagrams and coaching points in the back of the book, and you should do these at the end of the workout to cool down and relax.

Your warm-ups are integrated into the workouts to slowly increase heart rate and get the muscles warm. They have to be specific to the activity. For example cycling for ten minutes will not prepare your body for performing bicep curls with dumbbells. However performing two sets of bicep curls with a light resistance will prepare your biceps for the heavier resistance that you are about to lift as part of your workout. So the workouts are designed to integrate these ideas. This also helps to keep your workout short. If however you are feeling stiff some mornings, you can do some mobility exercises. This is very simple and is done by simply moving the joint through its range of motion several times with no resistance. This is the same for all the joints (see diagram below for example of shoulder mobility exercise).

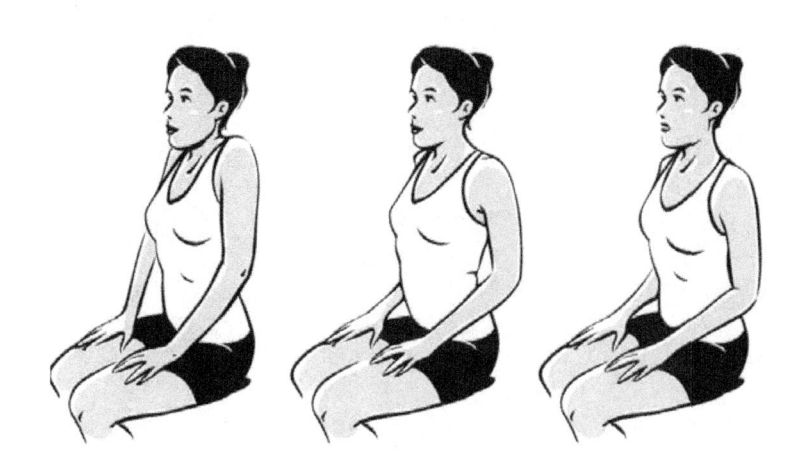

Perform ten full movements for any particular joint that is feeling stiff, or to all the joints: knees, shoulders, wrists, etc as a general mobility section. This helps to improve the lubrication of the joint by increasing the flow of synovial fluid within that joint. This will help to loosen up the joint until they are feeling freely movable. It is like adding oil to a squeaky chain. So any area that is feeling stiff, follow this pattern of limbering up and it will help.

This concludes the exercise plan. So now you are ready to begin. In the forthcoming chapters you will find information on types of exercises and diagrams etc. so it is important to read those. But you have now gained all the information that you need on food and exercise, and you know all of the truths so you are now ready to achieve *'the body you want'* It is important now to get started. You have taken the first step. You have found this book and that is the hardest step. Now you know the answers it is simply a matter of time and of course effort. But I know you can do it. I know you have always been willing to put the effort in, you just wanted to see results without having to starve yourself or spend two hours in a gym. Well you have now achieved that knowledge, and I know you can put in the effort. When you see the results, I know that you will pick up momentum and there will be no stopping you. This is where you become so important because you can now become someone else's angel. Inform, tell, offer advice to all those people struggling and battling with food, and dragging themselves through marathon gym workouts and over exertion. You know the truth now and you can help to spread the word. Kick out quick fixes and gimmicks and let the truth be made available to everybody, and then we can all get the '*body we want*' and the body we deserve.

Chapter 8

Progress sheet for resistance training

Resistance Workout:

Date:_____ Week:_____

Body Part	Exercise	Set	Kg day 1	2	3	reps day 1	2	3	Adj. day 1	2	3
Chest		1									
		2									
		3									
		4									
Back		5									
		6									
		7									
		8									
Shoulders		9									
		10									
		11									
		12									
Front arms Biceps		13									
		14									
		15									
		16									
Back arms Triceps		17									
		18									
		19									
		20									
Legs		21									
		22									
		23									
		24									
Mid section Abdominals		25									
		26									
		27									
		28									

Chapter 9

Exercise lists and instruction

<u>Chest</u>

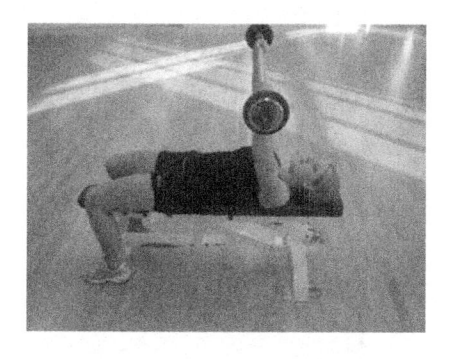

Bench Press
- Begin by lying on the bench
- Hands just wide of shoulder width
- The bar should be above the chest

- Feet flat on the floor
- Back flat on the bench
- Slowly lower the bar under control until it touches chest
- This should take 2 seconds
- Then lift the bar back to the start position in a controlled manner
- Keep weight above elbows

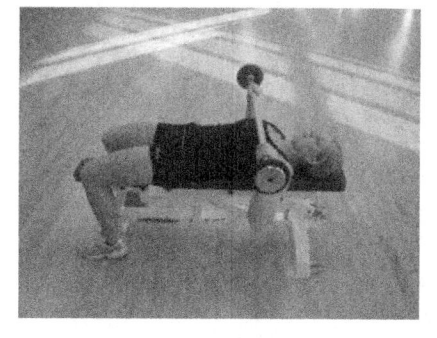

Dumbbell Press

- Starting position is the same

- As you lower the weights keep your forearm vertical so that the weight remains above the elbow

- Lower in a controlled manner as before, taking 2 seconds

- Stop when you reach a 90° at the elbow or when the dumbbells reach chest height.

- Return to start position slowly

- Tins, water bottles etc can be used

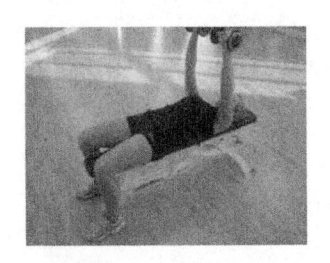

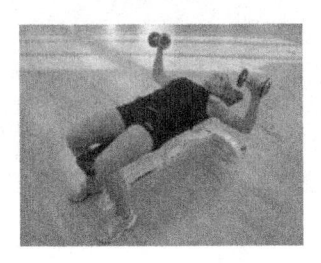

Dumbbell Flyes

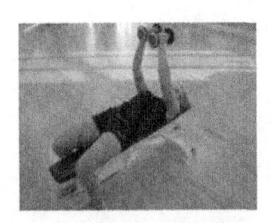

- Begin with the dumbbells above the chest

- Arms should be almost straight but maintain a slight bend to keep pressure off the elbow joint

- Slowly lower the dumbbells out to the side until they reach a horizontal position across from the chest

- This should take 2 seconds then return to the start position and repeat

Press-ups
- Begin with hands just wide of shoulder width and knees on ground

- Bend the elbows to lower chest down and forward towards the ground

- Stop when elbows reach 90° angle

- Take 2 seconds to lower and then return to the start position in a controlled way

- To make this easier brings knees closer to hips, or more difficult by having legs straight and knees off the ground

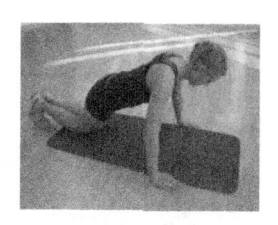

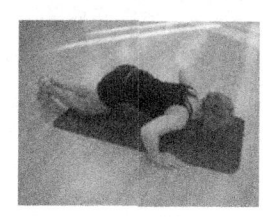

Press-ups using ball
- The hand position is the same is above

- The legs should begin on the ball

- The difficulty depends on the positioning of the ball. The closer to the hips the easier the exercise, and towards the feet is more difficult.

- Continue as above lowering and lifting in a controlled manner

- Only lower until elbows reach a 90°

Back

Single arm row

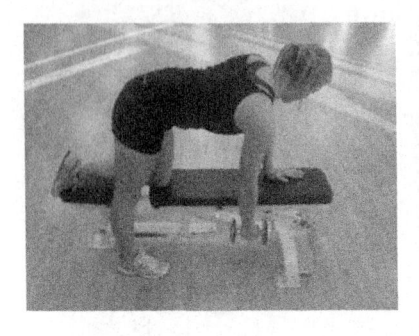

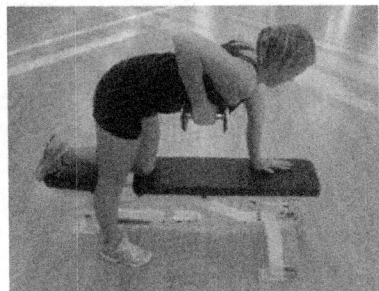

- Start position is important as you need to ensure that you have a straight back position and a stable base.

- Ensure body weight is supported on bench through knee and hand evenly and that the standing foot gives balance.

- Start with hand below the shoulder holding the weight

- Pull up slowly until the dumbbell is underneath the arm pit

- Keep the elbow high and the weight close to the body

- Slowly lower back to the start position

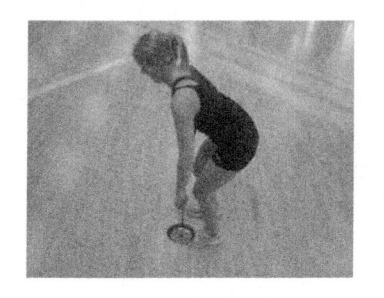

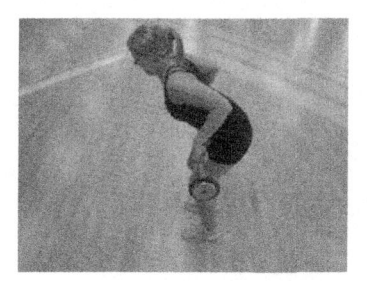

Barbell Row

- Start with feet shoulder width apart
- Hold bar with an over hand grip
- Hands shoulder width apart
- Have knees bent and back straight
- Bend forward so that you have room to pull the weight past the knees
- Pull shoulder blades together and pull the weight up to stomach
- Keep the speed slow and controlled
- Pause for a second in this position
- Slowly lower back to the start position
- Maintain straight back throughout this movement

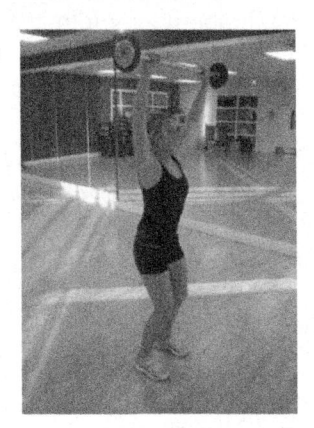

Shoulders

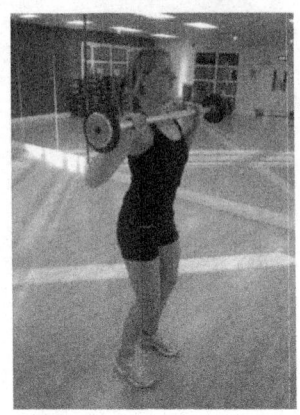

Shoulder Press Bar

- Begin with feet shoulder width apart
- Have a slight bend in the knees
- Hold the bar just wide of shoulder width so that you have your hands above your elbows. The bar can rest on your collar.
- As you begin to push the bar above your head keep your hands above the elbows
- Press until you have straightened your arms fully but do not lock out the elbow, keep it soft on the joints
- Try not to pause at the top just proceed to lower again slowly back to the start position and repeat.

Dumbbell shoulder press

- The starting position for this exercise is the same as with the barbell

- Position each dumbbell so that the hands are directly above the elbows and the forearms are vertical

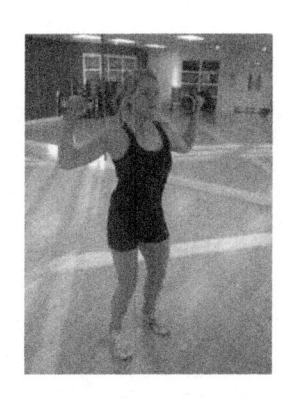

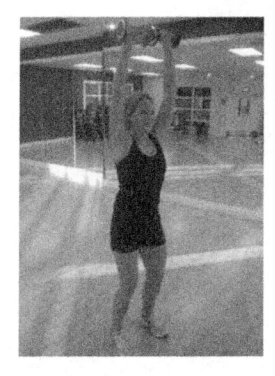

- Press the arms straight until the dumbbells meet above your head

- Again do not lock out the arms, keep the movement soft on the joints

- Try not to pause at the top as before

Upright Row

- Begin with feet shoulder width apart and knees slightly bent holding the dumbbells in front of the body

- Keep the dumbbells together as if they were joined

- Lead the pull upwards with the elbows and they will remain above the wrists throughout the movement

- Pull upwards until the dumbbells are just about chest high and then without pausing slowly lower back to the start position in a controlled way

- Keep the back straight throughout and the weights close to the body

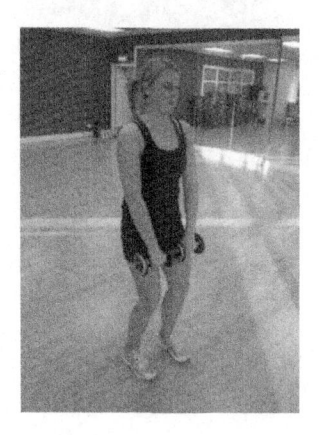

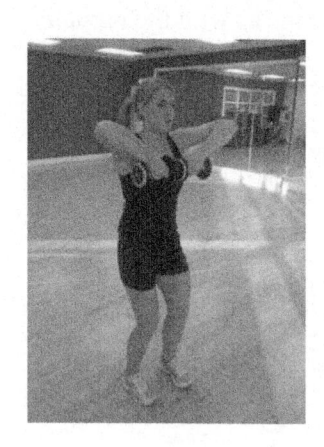

Lateral Raise

- Begin with feet shoulder width apart and knees slightly bent

- Hold the dumbbells at your side

- Maintain a very slight bend in the elbow throughout the movement

- Lift to the side until the dumbbells are shoulder high keeping back straight

- Turn the dumbbells slightly forward as if pouring water out of a bottle

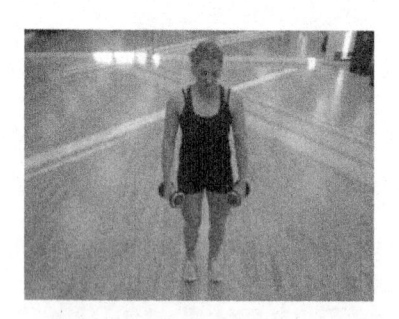

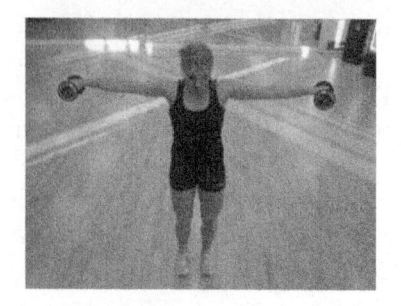

- Do not pause at the top or the bottom of the movement make it continuous
- Return back to the start position in a slow and controlled manner

Dumbbell Front Raise

- Begin with feet shoulder width apart, knees bent and back straight
- Hold dumbbells in front of the thighs and next to each other
- Keep back straight and slowly lift the dumbbells forward and upwards until they reach shoulder height
- Then slowly lower back to start position in a controlled manner
- When performing this lift do not swing the weight up, use your shoulder muscles to lift in a controlled manner maintaining a straight back position

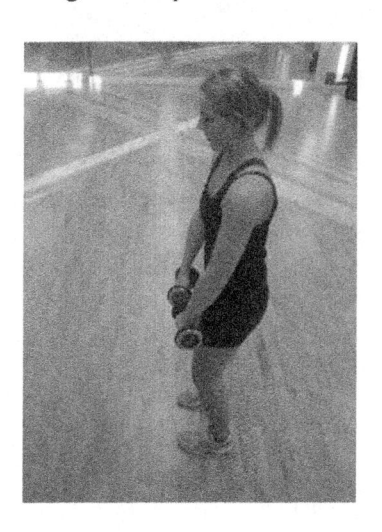

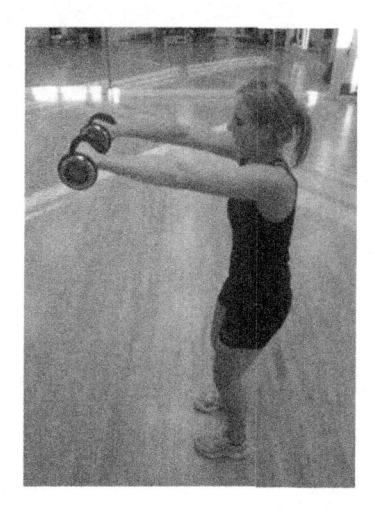

Biceps

Dumbbell Bicep Curl

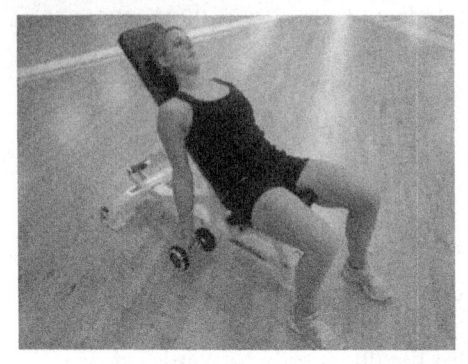

- Begin seated on an inclined bench position
- Have arms hanging by your side holding the weights
- Maintain this arm position and then bend the elbow to lift the weight until the arm is bent to at least 90°
- Then lower slowly and controlled back to the start position
- Keep your back in the seat supported throughout

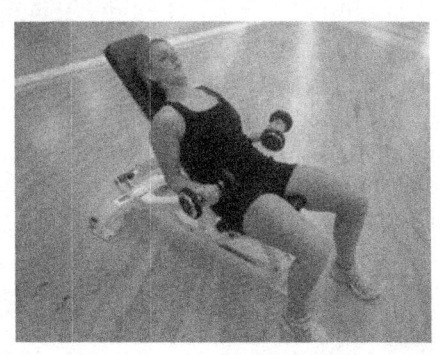

Barbell Bicep Curl

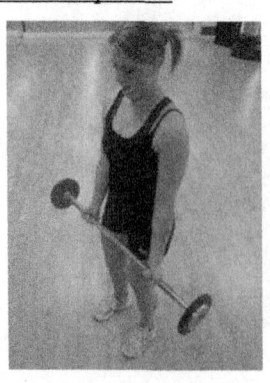

- Begin with feet shoulder width apart, knees slightly bent and back straight
- Hold the bar with an underhand grip
- Hands holding the bar about shoulder width apart
- Begin with arms straight and then curl the bar up until the elbow passes through a 90° angle

- Keep the elbows fixed by your side and keep the back straight throughout this movement

- Do not swing the bar up, use the bicep to lift the weight

- Slowly return to the start position in a controlled manner

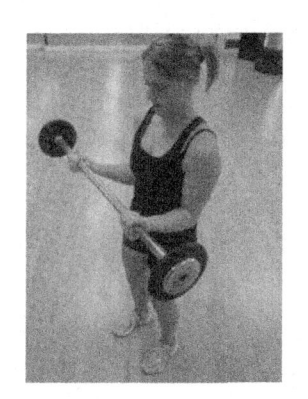

Triceps

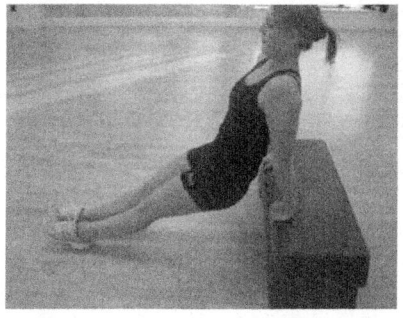

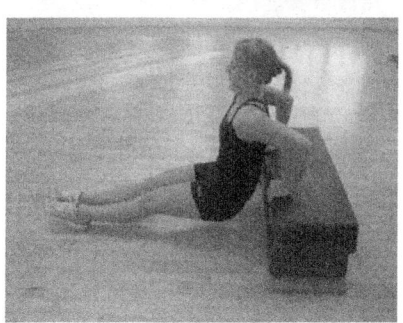

Tricep Dips

- Start with fingers pointing forward and hanging over the front of the step, legs straight and bum close to the front of the step

- Arms begin in a straight position

- From here bend the elbow to 90° lowering towards the floor

- Then push down and lift your body back to the start position

- Perform this movement in a controlled manner

- If this is too hard you can do the alternative below

- In this case you start with a bent leg position, this makes it easier because you can take some of your body weight with your legs

- If you want to make this movement more difficult for a progression you can attempt this with your feet raised onto a box or step or even the ball.

- This means that more of your body weight is forced onto your arms

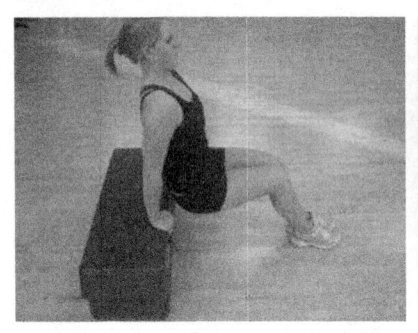

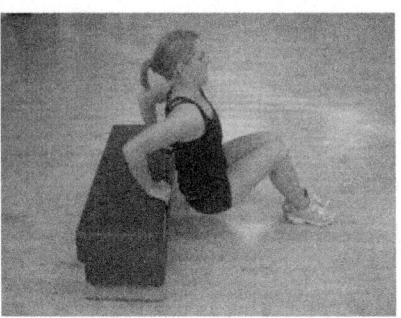

Lying Barbell Extensions

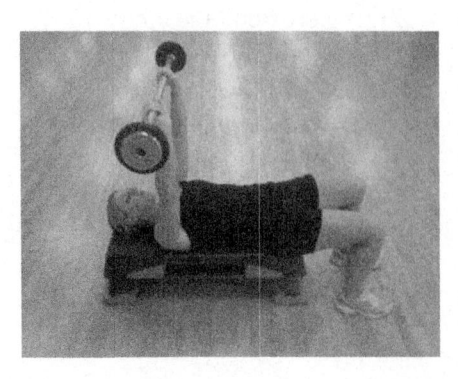

- Begin by lying on a bench or step holding the bar above your shoulders

- Hold the bar with hands shoulder width apart in an over hand position

- Bend the elbow so that you slowly lower the bar towards your head

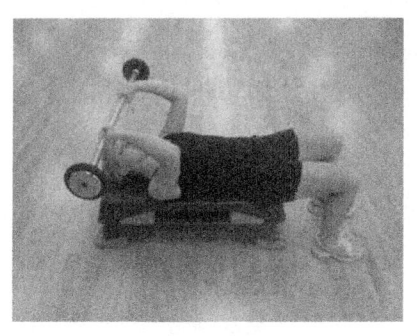

- Keep your shoulders firm so that you only move the forearm not the total arm

- Lower and lift back to start position in a slow and controlled manner

- Do not pause at the top or bottom of the movement

Dumbbell Kickbacks
- Begin with one hand and one knee on the bench supporting your body weight

- The position should give you a maintained straight back position whilst the other leg should give you balance by standing on the floor

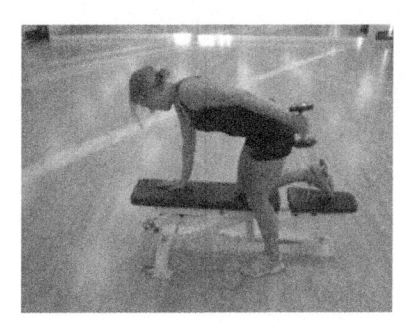

- Start with your arm in a right angle position by your side with the dumbbell facing the ground

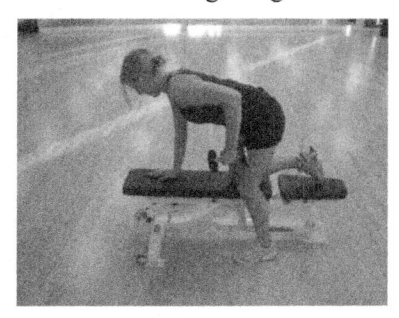

- Then extend the arm so that the dumbbell lifts backwards and your arm becomes straight

- Slowly lower back to the start position

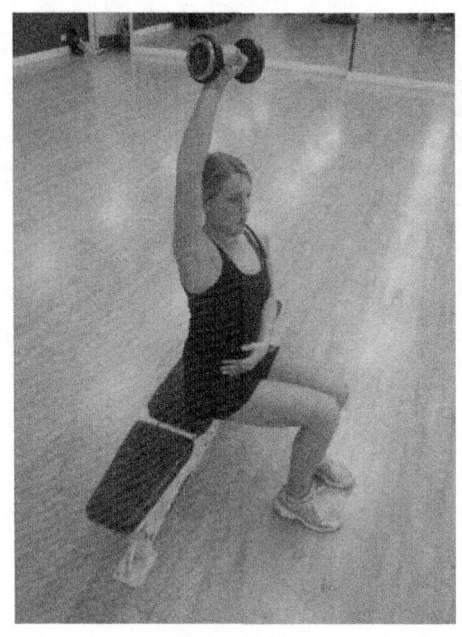

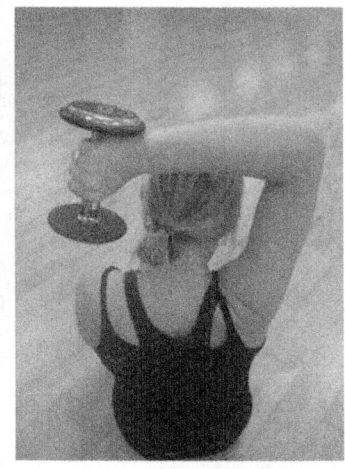

Single Arm Extensions

- Begin by sitting down or standing up

- Take hold of the dumbbell and straighten arm above your head

- Your arm can actually use your head as a guide for the position

- Then slowly bend your arm at the elbow until the dumbbell lowers behind your head

- Do this carefully to protect yourself and begin with a light weight to practice this movement

- From here straighten your arm back to the start position in a slow and controlled manner

- Try not to pause at the bottom or the top of the movement it should be slow and continuous

Legs

Lunges

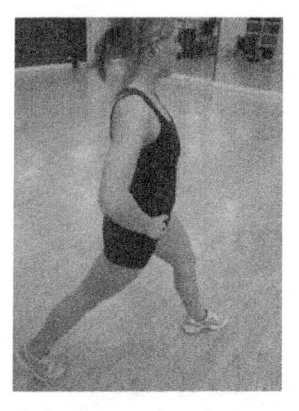

- Begin with one foot stretched out in front of the other
- Keep your back straight and your head up
- Place hands on your hips or holding onto weights
- Bend both knees to lower your body towards the ground
- Do not let your knee touch the ground but lower until you reach a right angle at each knee
- Keep your front knee from going in front of your toes as this places unnecessary pressure on your Achilles
- Return to the start position by pushing through your front heel

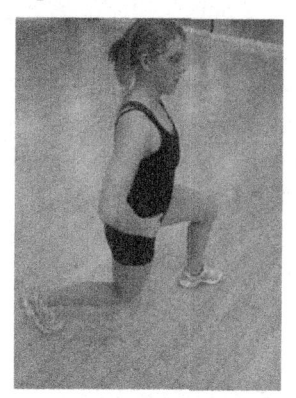

Squats

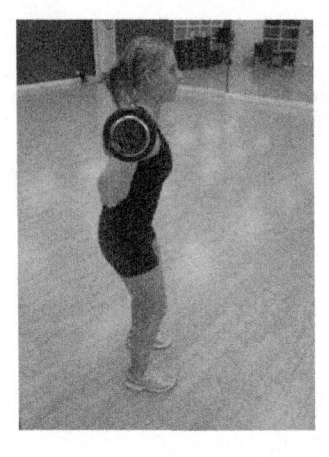

- Begin with feet shoulder width apart, back straight and head up
- Hold the bar on your shoulders or dumbbells by your side
- Bend your knees and stick your bum out behind you keeping your back straight and your head and chest up
- Keep your knees behind your toes and feet flat on the floor
- To return to the start position push heels through the floor and thrust your hips forward
- Maintain a straight back throughout

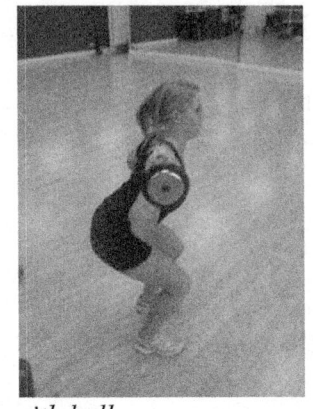

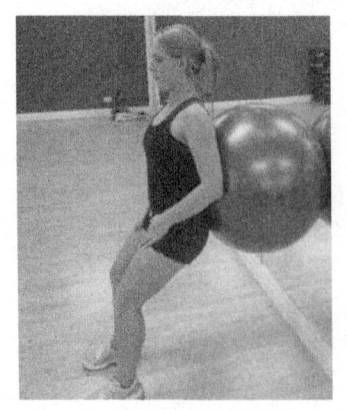

Squats with ball

- Place ball against a wall and position it on your lower back
- Angle your feet away from the wall slightly and keep feet shoulder width apart
- Keep back straight

- Bend legs and lower your body until you reach a 90° angle at your knees

- Slowly and steadily return to the standing position but do not pause at the top to gain rest, continue back into the squat

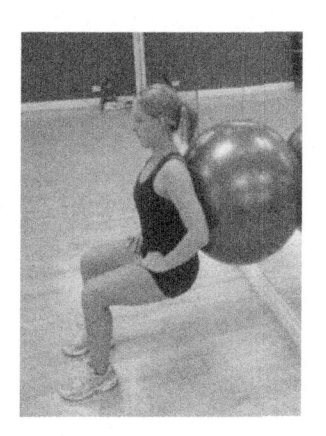

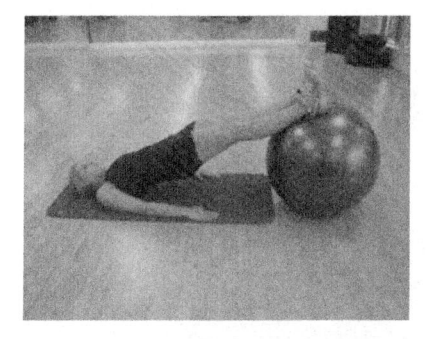

Leg Curl on ball

- Place feet on the ball

- Lift hips off the ground to make your body into a straight poistion from shoulders to feet

- Keep arms on the ground for balance

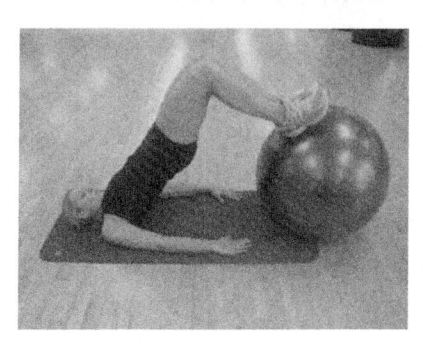

- From here bend your knees to a 90° angle

- Attempt to keep a straight position from shoulders to knees

- This will mean that your hips will lift higher as you bend your knees

- Then lower slowly back to the start position in a controlled manner

Basic Abdominal Crunch

- Lie back with your knees bent and your feet on the ground
- Find a neutral spine position so that you are not arching too far
- Place your hands on your chest or for more intensity by your temples as this adds more weight to the exercise
- Then crunch forward contracting your abdominal muscles a bit like when you cough or laugh and lift your shoulders off the ground
- Return back to the start position in a slow and controlled manner

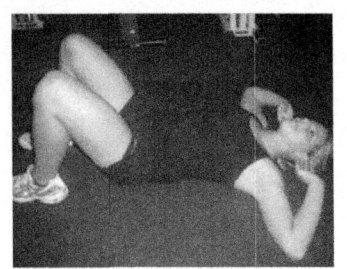

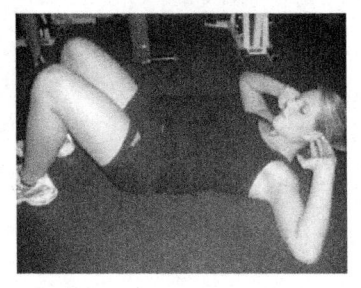

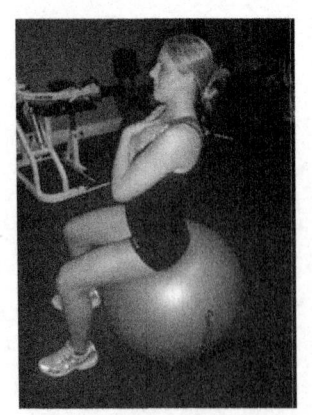

Crunch on ball

- Start by being seated towards the front of the ball
- Take some of your body weight on your feet and position your hands on your chest
- From here you will slowly lower yourself backwards contracting your abdominals as you do to control the movement

- You will end up almost lying back on the ball

- It is important to keep the ball still during this movement. Otherwise, if the ball rolls with you as you move, your abdominal muscles will relax and you will not get the benefit of the movement

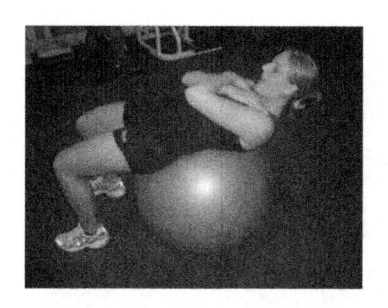

- Return to the start position by contracting again and sitting up

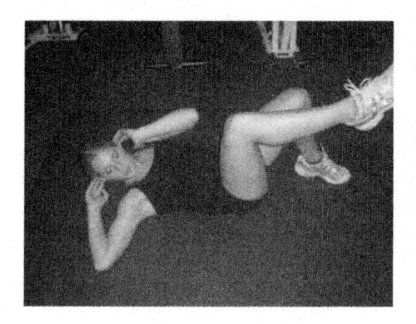

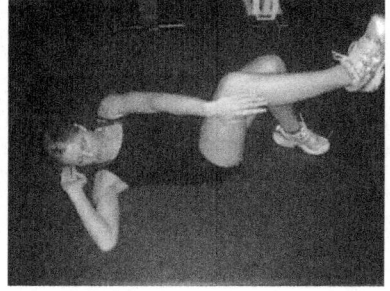

Twisting crunch

- Very similar to the basic crunch but this time one leg is to be lifted off the ground and the opposite shoulder will be lifted so that they come towards each other

- Then lower them both back to the ground in a slow and controlled manner and repeat on the opposite side of the body

Semi sit ups

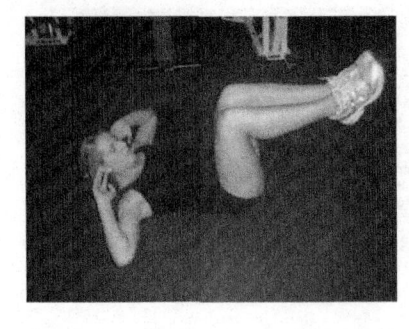

- This is the same as the basic crunch only this time your legs will be raised into right angles
- The legs are held fixed in this position throughout the crunch
- Lift and lower the shoulders as in the basic abdominal crunch

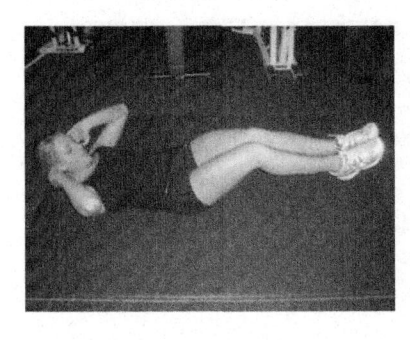

Double Crunch

- This time the upper body and legs are lifted in unison
- Perform this movement slowly and controlled throughout
- This takes some practice to balance on the glutes (bottom)

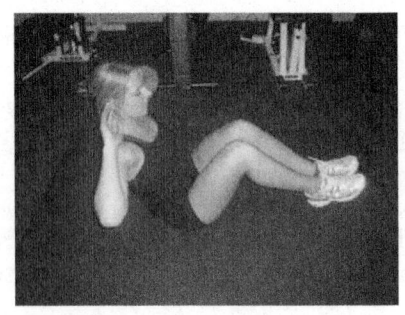

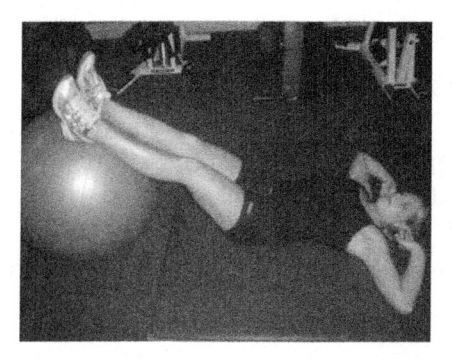

Crunch legs on ball

- In this exercise the ball is used to bring into use more core muscles

- The idea is that you keep the ball in a straight line backwards and forwards

- As you perform the basic crunch with your upper body you feet pull the ball towards you

- It is important to focus and concentrate on contracting your abdominals through this movement

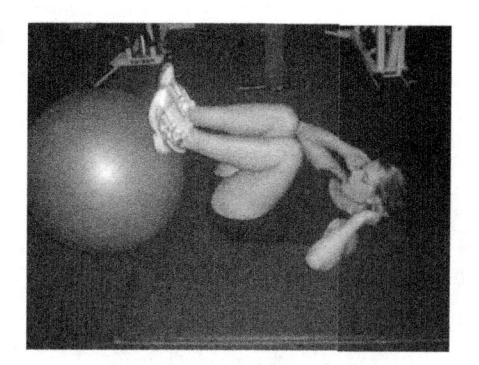

- Return back to the start position in a controlled manner

Twist crunch with ball

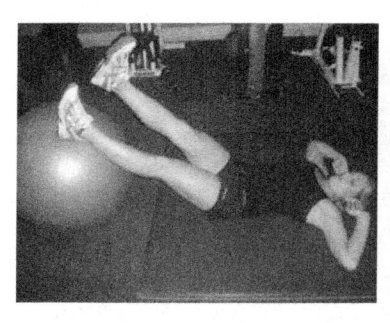

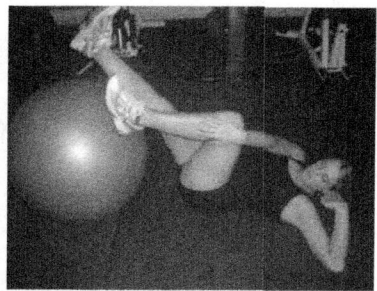

- This time have one foot on the ball

- The other leg remains almost straight held in the air
- The leg on the ball pulls the ball towards you
- At the same time you crunch the opposite shoulder off the ground and reach across to the leg pulling the ball
- Return to the start position in a slow and controlled manner
- Obviously you will repeat this on the same leg for a full set
- Then repeat with other leg on ball

Heel touches on ball

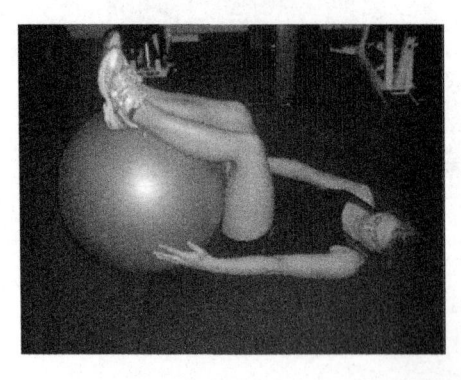

- Heels are placed on the ball and the ball is tucked close to the thighs
- Hold the ball in a fixed position and crunch your shoulders slightly off the ground
- From here you will reach sideways until you can reach the centre of the ball and then reach back to the centre and back across to the other side
- This will work predominantly in a lateral movement

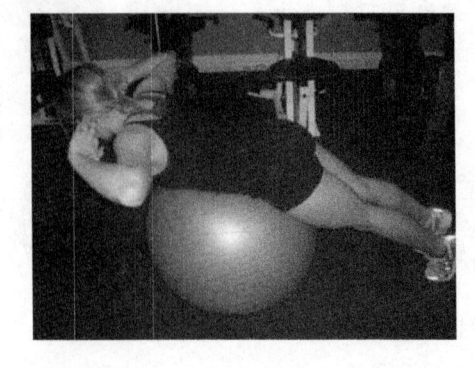

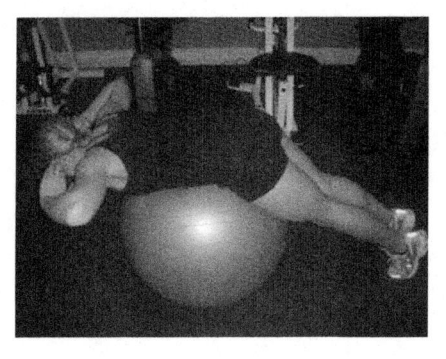

Lower back raise using ball

- Begin by positioning the ball underneath your stomach/pelvis
- Have your legs straight and feet on the ground for stability
- Place your hands by your head
- Begin from a relaxed spine position and move to a straight spine position by tensing the muscles in the lower back
- Do not lift too far and hyperextend or go further than a horizontal position in your back
- Slowly lower back to the start position in a controlled manner

Stretches

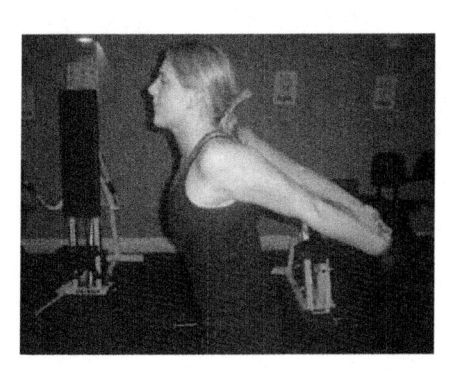

Chest stretch

- Put your hands together behind your back
- Lift up until you feel the stretch through the front of your shoulders and chest
- Hold for 30 seconds

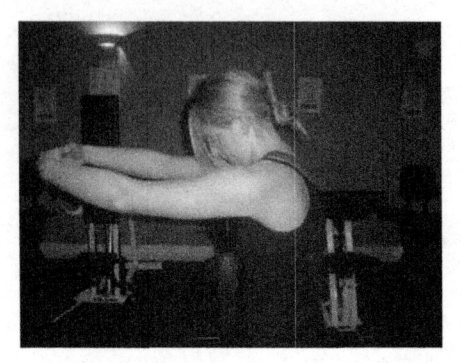

Upper back stretch

- Link hsnds in front of your chest and arch your back forwards
- Feel the stretch through your upper back muscles

Shoulder stretch

- Take one arm across your body midline as shown
- Hold it with your free arm and apply a little pressure
- Pulling the arm away from its origin

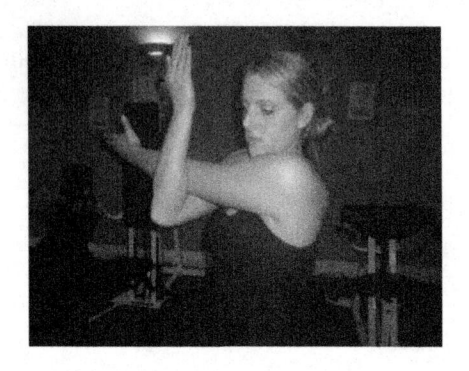

Tricep Stretch

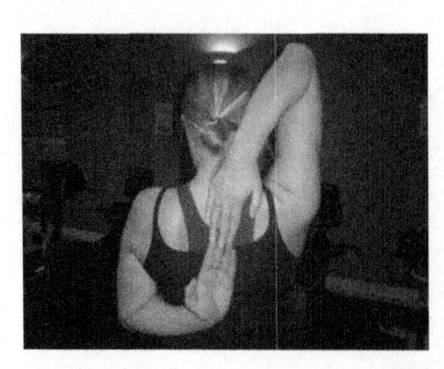

- As you can see this can require some flexibility
- Do your best to link hands behind your back
- This will aid the stretch
- If you cannot do this use the free hand to push the top elbow behind your back

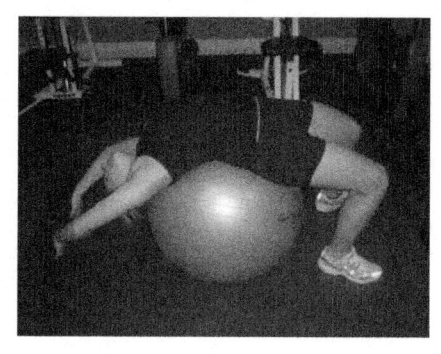

Abdominal Stretch

- Relax over the ball in this manner
- This position gives a natural stretch of the abdominals
- You can relax in this position
- Use your feet and hands for balance

Thigh Stretch

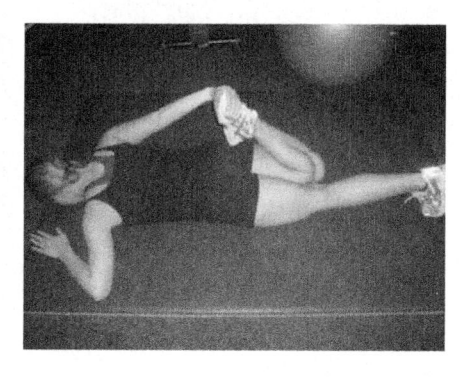

- Begin by lying on your front
- Bend one leg and take hold of the ankle with free hand
- By pulling back on the ankle and tilting your pelvis forward into the ground you will feel your thigh stretching

Calf Stretch

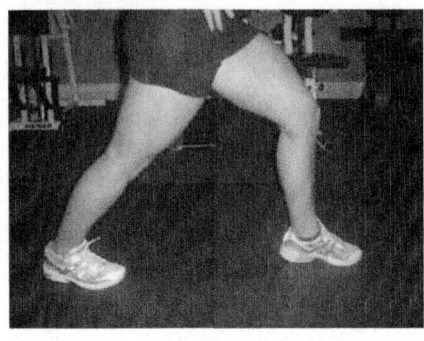

- Place one foot in front of the other
- Keep your heels pushed into the ground
- Lean forward and push through the heel of the back leg
- This is the leg that you will feel the calf stretching

Hamstring Stretch (Back thigh)

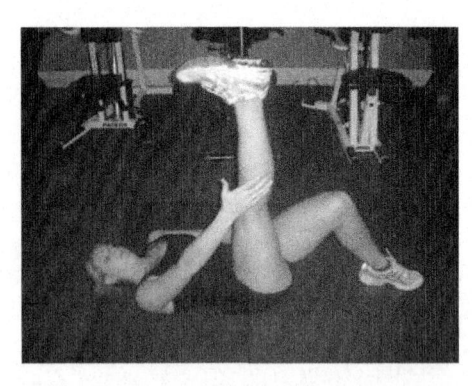

- Lie on your back and place one foot on the ground
- Hold your other leg behind the knee and straighten your leg
- Pull the leg towards you until you feel a stretch at the back of the thigh
- Hold this position for thirty seconds

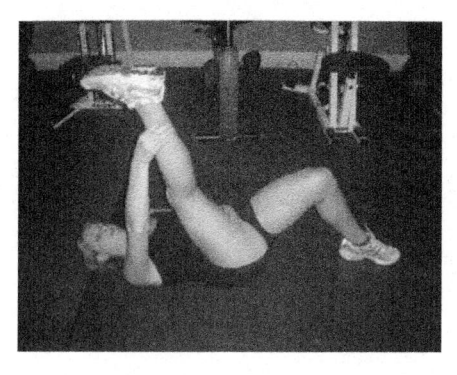

- This demonstrates the position of the stretch when the hamstrings or back of thigh are more flexible

- Try to keep your bottom on the ground when you are pulling leg backwards

- This ensures that the hamstrings are being stretched and that it is not just the pelvis lifting off the ground

- With all stretches be careful to hold the position fixed do not bounce or attempt to push too far

- Hold the stretch for 30 seconds

- Relax and repeat if necessary

- Each time attempting to push just to the point you feel the stretch

Exercise lists

I mentioned earlier that you can exercise at home or in the gym and I have given examples of exercises that you can use anywhere. However there are many more exercises that are available. I have compiled a list below for each muscle group, some of which you will recognize and others you will find are machines found in gyms. I will not be describing these exercises to you because the machines may differ slightly in each gym. However if you do use them in the format explained in the training plan they will have the same desired effect.

Use these lists to select your daily routine for the resistance training plan. Remember you can choose a different exercise each day.

Chest

Bench Press
Dumbbell Press
Flyes
Press Ups
Ball Press Ups
Machine Chest Press
Machine Flyes/Pec dec

Back

Single arm row
Barbell row
Lat Pull down
Machine row
Cable row

Shoulders

Shoulder Press Bar
Shoulder Press Dumbbells
Shoulder Press Machine
Upright row
Lateral raise
Front raise

Biceps

Dumbbell curl
Barbell curl
Preacher curl machine
Standing dumbbell curls
Concentration curl

Triceps

Dips
Barbell extensions
French press
Tricep pushdowns-cable machine
Single arm extension
Kickbacks

Legs

Lunges
Squats
Ball squats
Leg curl using ball
Leg press machine
Leg extension machine
Leg curl machine

Chapter 10

Meal ideas and portion amounts

Meal 1

Daily intake:

- ❖ Carbohydrates   2 servings
- ❖ Protein   1 serving
- ❖ Vegetables   2 servings

You will need:

1 Tomato, ½ Green pepper, ½ Red onion, 75-100g Skinless Chicken Breast, 4tbsp Brown rice, Selected leaves.
Seasoning; Paprika, Chilli, Parsley, Pepper.

Preparation:

1. Chop onion, pepper, tomato finely and heat in pan until desired consistency.
2. Season chicken breast and grill until cooked through.
3. Boil brown rice.

Serving:

Place chicken on top of rice, pour tomato, onion and pepper sauce on top and garnish with leaves.

Meal 2

Daily intake:

- Carbohydrates   0 servings
- Protein   2 serving
- Vegetables   2 servings

You will need:
100-150g Cod (or other white fish), 100g tinned green lentils, 6 cherry tomatoes skinned, olive oil, ½ clove garlic, 1 stick celery, ½ leek, ½ onion.
Seasoning: Thyme and Parsley

Preparation:
1. Steam the cod for 15-20 minutes
2. Heat olive oil and add finely chopped onion
3. Add the garlic, celery and leek and cook for 3 minutes
4. Add lentils, tomatoes and seasoning and cook for further 3 minutes

Serving:
Spoon the lentil and tomato mixture onto a plate and lie the fish on top seasoning to desired taste

Meal 3

Daily Intake:
- Carbohydrates   2 servings
- Protein   1 serving
- Vegetables   2 servings

You will need:
100g skinless cubed chicken breast, ½ red pepper, ½ yellow pepper, 6 cherry tomatoes, 4tbsp brown rice

Seasoning: Balsamic vinegar, thyme, olive oil, chicken stock

Preparation:
1. Mix the seasoning marinade in a bowl using all of the seasoning ingredients
2. Pour the marinade over the cubed chicken and vegetables
3. Thread vegetables and chicken onto kebab skewers
4. Grill for 12 minutes or until cooked through, turning regularly

Serving:
Place the rice on a plate and position the skewers on the top and serve immediately

Meal 4

Daily intake:
- Carbohydrates   2 servings
- Protein   1 serving
- Vegetables   1 serving

You will need:
2 pieces of whole-meal bread, 50g cottage cheese, rocket leaves, cranberry sauce, 1 tomato

Preparation:
1. Spread the cranberry sauce onto the 2 slices of bread
2. Mix the cottage cheese with the rocket and spread onto the cranberry sauce
3. Slice the tomato and lay on top
4. Chop simple sandwich in half (simple and tasty)

Chapter 11

Vitamin and mineral sources and uses in within the body

Vitamin B1 (Thiamin):

Use in the body: Helps to release energy from carbohydrates during metabolism. It is Important for health of nerves and muscles including the heart. It helps to prevent fatigue and irritability.

Source: Pork, whole grains, dried beans and peas, sunflower seeds, nuts.

Vitamin B2 (Riboflavin):

Use in the body: Helps to metabolize carbohydrates, fat and protein to release energy. Supports good vision and healthy hair, skin and nails. Necessary for normal cell growth.

Source: Liver and other organ meats, poultry, fish, dried peas and beans, nuts, sunflower seeds, cheese, eggs, yogurt, milk, whole grains, green leafy vegetables.

Vitamin B3 (niacin, nicotinic acid, nicotinamide):

Use in the body: Important for healthy skin and digestive tract tissue. It stimulates circulation. Energy metabolism.

Source: Liver and other organ meats, veal, pork, poultry, fish, nuts, dried beans, dried fruit, green leafy vegetables, whole grains, milk, eggs.

Vitamin B5 (Pantothenic acid):

Use in the body: Important in energy production and utilisation. It supports adrenal glands to increase production of hormones to counteract stress. Important for healthy skin and nerves.

Source: Nuts, beans, seeds, dark green leafy vegetables, poultry, dried fruit, milk.

Vitamin B6 (Pyridoxine):

Use in the body: Helps body protein to build body tissue and in metabolism of fat. Facilitates the release of glycogen from liver and muscles. Helps in red blood cell production.

Source: Sunflower seeds, beans, poultry, liver, eggs, nuts, bananas, dried fruit, green leafy vegetable.

Vitamin B12 (Cyanocobalamin):

Use in the body: Important in formation of red blood cells and building genetic material. Stimulates growth in children. Helps functioning of nervous system. Metabolism of protein and fat in the body.

Source: Animal protein foods, including meat, fish, shellfish, poultry, milk, yogurt, eggs.

Folate (folic acid, Folacin):

Use in the body: Helps form red blood cells. Essential during pregnancy for its importance in cell division. Supports brain functions.

Source: Dark green leafy vegetable, nuts, beans, whole grains, fruit, fruit juices, liver, egg yolks.

Vitamin C (Ascorbic Acid):

Use in the body: essential for connective tissue found in skin, cartilage, bones, and teeth. Helps heal wounds. Antioxidant. Stimulates immune system. Aids in absorption of iron.

Source: Citrus fruit, berries, melons, dark green vegetables, cauliflower, tomatoes, green and red peppers, cabbage, potatoes.

Vitamin A (Retinol):

Use in the body: Tissue maintenance. Healthy skin, hair, and mucous membranes. Helps us to see in dim light. Essential for normal growth and reproduction.

Source: Liver, deep yellow, orange and dark green leafy vegetables and fruits. Cheese, milk, fortified margarine.

Vitamin D3 (cholecalciferol):

Use in the body: Helps to regulate calcium metabolism and bone calcification.

Source: Fortified and full fat dairy products, tuna, salmon, cod liver oil.

Vitamin E (D-alpha-tocopherol):

Use in the body: Antioxidant to prevent cell membrane damage.

Source: Vegetable oils, nuts, seeds, fish, whole grains, green leafy vegetables.

Vitamin K (Phylloquinone):

Use in the body: Necessary for normal blood clotting.

Source: Dark green leafy vegetable, cabbage.

Calcium:

Use within the body: essential for strength of bones and teeth.

Source: Milk products, vegetables, sardines, clams and oysters.

Phosphorus:

Use within the body: A component of every cell including DNA, RNA and ATP.

Source: Whole grain cereals, egg yolks, fish, milk, meat, poultry, legumes, nuts.

Magnesium:

Use within the body: Activator of enzymes.

Source: Green vegetables, legumes, nuts, whole grain cereal, nuts, meat, chocolate.

Sodium:

Use within the body: Regulates fluid levels, involved in muscular contraction.

Source: Common table salt, and most foods except fruit.

Chlorine:

Use within the body: A component of digestive fluids and functions in combination with sodium.

Source: Table salt, meat, seafood, eggs, milk.

Potassium:

Use within the body: Involved in protein and carbohydrate metabolism.

Source: Meat, milk, cereals, vegetables, fruits, legumes.

Printed in Great Britain
by Amazon